T022148

KT-548-146

OF01032

Books should be returned to the SDH Library on or before
the date stamped above unless a renewal has been arranged

Salisbury District Hospital Library

Telephone: Salisbury (01722) 336262 extn. 4432 / 33

Out of hours answer machine in operation

MEN'S HEALTH – HOW TO DO IT

Edited by
DAVID CONRAD
and
ALAN WHITE

Foreword by
IAN BANKS

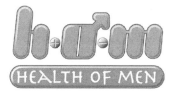

Radcliffe Publishing
Oxford • New York

Radcliffe Publishing Ltd
18 Marcham Road
Abingdon
Oxon OX14 1AA
United Kingdom

www.radcliffe-oxford.com
Electronic catalogue and worldwide online ordering facility.

British Library Cataloguing in Publication Data

A catalogue record for this book is available from the British Library.

ISBN-13 978 1 84619 192 3

Typeset by Egan Reid, Auckland, New Zealand
Printed and bound by TJI Digital, Padstow, Cornwall, UK

CONTENTS

Foreword

RHETORIC TO REALITY: DIRTY HANDS

There is a pecking order of activity in men's health. Fine words are not in short supply, particularly those addressing inequalities sentencing men to an early death. Fine deeds are less easy to find, rhetoric is always cheaper than action but unfortunately many initiatives just 'seemed like a good idea at the time'. As an issue men's health is plagued by myth, ignorance and inequality, but most of all by a lack of solid research based on evidence-based work with men themselves. Lofty academics pontificate endlessly on the meaning of 'masculinity' yet never get their invariably white Caucasian, middle class hands dirty on what really impacts on Y chromosome owners. In truth, men should not be expected to self-destruct like some Mission Impossible tape. Yet a Glasgow man will live around ten years less than a Dorset prostate comrade. Suicide amongst young men with its huge predominance amongst low income groups is not just a tragedy, it is national disgrace. Male late presentation with life-threatening conditions is accepted throughout the medical profession despite a lack of fundamental research to confirm, let alone address, the problem. Meanwhile the health of men, women and children suffer. If there is anything we have learned it is that the health and wellbeing of both sexes is often inextricably linked. Perhaps the Equality Act, in force April 2007, placing for the first time emphasis on equitable outcomes based on gender, might just bring minds to bear.

The Bradford team didn't just wonder about masculinity and scratch male pattern baldness, they did something measurable about men's health and ethnicity so other workers could use their evidence base to actually change the dreadful health status quo.

Welcome to the Bradford Health of Men's guide on how to do it. An excellent and unique 'Dirty Hands Manual'.

Ian Banks
President
Men's Health Forum
February 2007

Preface

Based on the award-winning work of the Bradford Health of Men (HoM) Services, this book is for anyone who wants to find out how to successfully set up and deliver health services aimed at men and boys. Traditionally, men have been seen as reluctant to access health services, but getting men to engage with their health isn't an impossible task once you're equipped with a few tricks of the trade.

Part One gives an overview of the Bradford HoM project and essential introductions to men's health and health promotion, setting out why there's a need for this kind of work and what it broadly aims to achieve.

Part Two is comprised of nine practical chapters on establishing different kinds of services to meet the health needs of men and boys. Each is based on successful HoM projects and written by people who delivered those projects on the ground. Throughout this section you'll come across 'Info', 'Handy Hint' and 'Warning' boxes giving key information, practical tips and things to watch out for. Although the sample of HoM services covered is quite broad, there are common core principles which are emphasised throughout the book and which you can easily apply to devise projects of your own.

Part Three includes a personal account of how HoM came into being, a discussion on what it takes to be a men's health worker and reflections from the team on some of their less successful moments!

Although this is primarily intended to be a practical guide for practitioners, much of the book will also be of interest to academics, policy makers and managers charged with implementing the new Gender Duty, demonstrating what can be achieved with adequate resources, a flexible approach and a sound understanding of men's needs.

David Conrad and Alan White
February 2007

About the editors

David Conrad MA, MSc

David has worked as a researcher at the Centre for Men's Health since completing an MSc in Public Health in 2005. As well as working on the study of men's usage of the HoM services, he has written papers on the sociology of the body, defining social capital and art in health.

Professor Alan White

Alan was the world's first professor of Men's Health. He has created a Centre for Men's Health at Leeds Metropolitan University, which is a focus for research and education on the health of men. He is founder member of the Men's Health Forum (England and Wales) and the Chair of the Board of Trustees since 2000.

His research includes a *Scoping Study on Men's Health* for the Department of Health in 2001, a report on the *State of Men's Health* across 17 European Countries (for the European Men's Health Forum) which was launched at the European Parliament in 2003, and he has recently completed a study into the *Patterns of Mortality for Young Men and Women (aged 15–44 years) Across 44 Countries*. Other on-going research includes the study of men's usage of the Bradford Health of Men Services and the evaluation of *Self Care for People* and *Self Care for Primary Health Care Professionals* as part of the National Working in Partnership Programme of work. Alan's work also includes a needs based analysis of men who received brachytherapy or external beam therapy for prostate cancer.

About the contributors

Chris Bradley RN, BSc
Chris is a men's health nurse at Airedale Primary Care Trust (PCT). As well as working on a range of projects with the HoM team, he established and currently delivers erectile dysfunction and male incontinence clinics based in health centres:

> I disliked school – never recovered from moving to the comprehensive system. I was a bit of a loner. I did the daredevil stuff trying to impress – riding down our only local hill on my bike, climbing trees etc. When we were older we took much greater risks, learning to drive and ride motor bikes on local waste land in old wrecks, making pipe bombs from weed killer . . . the list was amazing. The only serious injuries we received were from each other.
>
> I somehow managed to survive to adulthood. I have five children, three by my first marriage, now grown up with children of their own, and two very young children with my wife of 12 years, whom I met when I started nurse training at 39 years old.
>
> Men's health was a natural area for me to work in. I lived it, lost loved ones, mistreated others and myself and can see how small changes can make huge differences.
>
> My school experience put me off academic study for many years so I only do courses that genuinely impact on improving my practice. I was therefore pleased to train as a nurse and achieve my degree through modular study. My chapter in this book is drawn straight from experience; it is designed to start the debate, rather than provide a set of concrete answers.

Ruth Cross RN, BSc (Hons), MSc, PGCHE
Ruth is Course Leader for the MSc Public Health – Health Promotion at Leeds Metropolitan University. She is a nurse by profession, with ten years of nursing experience in acute and emergency medicine and HIV/AIDS. She has a BSc in Health Psychology and an MSc in Health Education and Health Promotion. In addition to teaching on the MSc Public Health – Health Promotion course she teaches on a range of under/post graduate allied health professional and health related courses, including nursing, and is an active member of the Centre for Health Promotion Research at Leeds Metropolitan University.

Nick Davy RN

Nick qualified as a Registered Nurse in 1987 and has since worked in general medicine, oncology and terminal care both in England and abroad. He moved to Yorkshire in 1997 and worked in genitor-urinary medicine before starting to work in men's health in 2001. Through the men's health activities Nick became involved with Yorkshire MESMAC (one of the oldest and largest sexual health organisations in the country working with gay men, bisexual men and men who have sex with men) and has been a member of its Board of Trustees since 2004. He was a founding member of the BLAST project (Bradford Lads Against the Sex Trade), a group that has researched into and continues to support young men involved in and exploited through prostitution. Nick now coordinates the activities of Bradford City's men and boys health team and continues to have a strong interest in sexual health.

In his spare time Nick hopes one day to have climbed all the Munros (mountains over 3000 feet) in Scotland.

Andrew Harrison RN, BA, BSc (Hons)

Andrew embarked on a nursing career in Manchester and has worked in Accident and Emergency, Orthopaedics, Intensive Care and as a District Nurse/Team Leader. He joined HoM in 2002 and has thoroughly enjoyed the experiences to date.

In 2005 Andrew was awarded The Queen's Nursing Institute Innovation and Creative Practice Award for his work with men and weight management. He is currently studying for an MSc in Men's Health at Leeds Metropolitan University and is co-founder of a private initiative called *Men's Health Plus*.

Nigel Hughes RN, RSCN, BA (Hons), MA

Nigel has worked in health in both England and the USA for over 15 years. He is a trained nurse and health visitor and recently completed an MA in Public Health Leadership. He currently manages and leads on health improvement for Airedale PCT, Bradford and works as health inequalities lead for the West Yorkshire Strategic Health Authority two days per week. His interest in men's health developed over a number of years and led to his role as Chair of the HoM project.

Nigel has a keen interest in helping people to take control of their own health (self-care) and is currently leading a national self care project within the Bradford locality. The self care work has focussed on engaging with men within the workplace and is producing fantastic results. The challenge now is to ensure the delivery of this work on an industrial scale.

As for personal self care, Nigel supports Newcastle United, which does not help his mental wellbeing.

Mehzar Iqbal

Mehzar is a multilingual healthcare support worker for HoM, based at Airedale PCT. He speaks Urdu, Punjabi and Hindi and has played a key role in setting up and helping to deliver projects with ethnic minority communities across the Bradford and Airedale district, including successfully bringing men's health sessions into local mosques.

Dennis Jones BA (Hons), PGCE

Dennis currently works part time for the HoM project, concentrating on school work and, in 2006, men and mental wellbeing:

> After finishing a degree in Humanities in 1977 I worked as a meter reader in Derby, farmer and fisherman in the Orkney Islands, barman in Barcelona, window cleaner in Rotterdam and comic artist in Yorkshire. Subsequently I trained to be a teacher of English as a foreign language but used those skills to become a volunteer coordinator at MIND, the National Association for Mental Health, in 1984. There among other things I ran men's groups, developed advocacy progammes, worked with an art therapist and drama therapist and developed programmes to resettle long stay patients back into the community.
>
> Seven years later I joined the Health Promotion Service in Bradford as a specialist in sexual health. I continued men's health work by running a professional development day for regional health promotion people on men and health in 1993 and began the HoM group in 1998 with a group of male health visitors. Together we wrote the National Lottery bid that has funded the HoM project since 2003.
>
> The things I love most after my two daughters are t'ai chi, which I've been practising for 16 years and music – I play alto saxophone in a karaoke band and spent many years in community music bands. I performed in two of the four acts of a community opera which alternated the devising of the pieces between Huddersfield and Ogwara in Japan. I travelled to Japan to take part in the full performance in Ezuko Hall Theatre in Miyagi prefecture, in April 2006.

Merv Pemberton

Merv is employed as a healthcare support worker by Airedale PCT. He worked as a nursing assistant before joining the HoM team soon after the project started. Based on his own experiences of having been bullied at school, he devised an innovative and successful programme of anti-bullying intervention which has been delivered in schools, places of worship and other community venues. Along with his anti-bullying work, Merv has been involved in projects targeted towards the Afro-Caribbean community, as well as helping in the delivery of a range of other HoM services.

Martin Samangaya RN, BSc (Hons), MSc

Martin works as a Men's Health Advisor for Bradford and Airedale PCT. He is a registered nurse and an honorary Yorkshire lad with extensive experience of acute, primary and secondary nursing care. His particular area of interest is tackling inequalities in health, public health intervention and engaging with the hard to reach client groups. His thesis for his post graduate study was a quantitative study that looked at *Accessibility of Sexual Health Services for Young Men from Black and Minority Ethnic Groups Aged 16 to 25 Years Old*. Since coming into post Martin has been greatly involved in health related sessions at one of the housing projects for young people in Bradford, establishing a good working partnership with the young people and staff.

Martin once cycled to Genoa from England for three weeks with 25 other cyclists via the Alps as part of *Drop the Debt* campaign. He occasionally plays football and is a keen supporter of Altrincham Football Club.

Pete Westwood RN, BA (Hons)
Pete currently works for Bradford South and West PCT as a Public Health Practitioner (Men's Health), but has also worked in hospitals, as a District Nurse, within school nursing and as a smoking cessation specialist. He also spent a period as a nursing advisor on ITV's *Where The Heart Is*. He is currently studying at Leeds Metropolitan University for an MSc in Men's Health. Pete is co-founder of a private initiative called *Men's Health Plus*, which offers men's health services outside the NHS.

In his spare time Pete is a family man who tries to practice what he preaches regarding his health – to the point of completing a triathlon in 2005 to raise funds for a mental health charity.

Acknowledgements

The editors wish to acknowledge the contributions of the following people:

- Professor Keith Cash (for his work on the first phase of the study)
- Mike Worden (former HoM business coordinator)
- David Newman (current HoM business coordinator)
- Chris Andrew (HoM administrator)
- Jim Campbell (illustrator)

List of abbreviations

BME	black and minority ethnic
BMI	body mass index
BP	blood pressure
CO	carbon monoxide
CVD	cardiovascular disease
DoH	Department of Health
ED	erectile dysfunction
GP	general practitioner
GUM	genito-urinary medicine
HDA	Health Development Agency
HoM	Health of Men
IAG	Independent Advisory Group
MHF	Men's Health Forum
MSN	Microsoft Network
NEED	Nurse Education in Erectile Dysfunction
NHS	National Health Service
NRT	nicotine replacement product
Ofsted	Office for Standards in Education
PCT	primary care trust
PSHE	personal, social and health education
SEN	special educational needs
SRE	sex and relationships education
STI	sexually transmitted infection
TPU	Teenage Pregnancy Unit
TSE	testicular self-examination
WHO	World Health Organization

PART ONE

CHAPTER 1

Introduction

NIGEL HUGHES

THE BRADFORD MODEL

In 2002 Bradford was awarded a £1m grant from the New Opportunities Fund to set up a Healthy Living Centre based on men's health. The foundation of the grant application was the work being undertaken by the Bradford Health HoM key workers, a group of practitioners who had developed innovative men's health services for some of the hardest to reach groups in society.

This grant, with matched funding from the local trusts, enabled a cross-city programme of activities. At the time when the HoM project began, there were four primary care trusts (PCTs) in Bradford and Airedale which have now merged into a single trust, Bradford and Airedale Teaching PCT. Within each PCT there was one full-time key worker, part-funded by the *Big Lottery*. The Lottery also funded a 'half post' based within the Bradford District Public Health Partnership. Each PCT also provided additional support to the project as an 'in-kind' contribution. In one PCT this included two additional dedicated key workers. HoM is a cross-city initiative, with key workers originally being employed within one of the four PCTs, but having the ability to work across the city, sharing expertise and jointly setting up events.

HoM have delivered a broad range of projects, including projects in schools, work with the Youth Offending team, health drop-in sessions for homeless men, sexual health outreach work in male saunas, health-related pub quizzes, and health checks in workplaces and community settings known as health 'MOTs' (*see* Chapter 4). This book highlights the main principles for working effectively in this area by featuring a sample of some of the most successful projects, however the possibilities for delivering new types of innovative men's health services are essentially limitless.

Traditionally, health care has been delivered in clinics where the healthcare professionals have configured services for their own convenience. The expectation

3

is that the patient will learn to use the service and will conform to its structures and ways of working. Within the majority of the work of the HoM team there is a reversal of this expectation, with the team generally going into the men's environment and engaging with the men on their terms. This alters significantly the nature of the relationship that the team have with the men and the way the men use their services.

During the time that the HoM team have been working with funding from the *Big Lottery Fund,* researchers from the Centre for Men's Health at Leeds Metropolitan University have been exploring with the team and with the men who use their services the decision making that men go through in choosing to attend. The intention of the study was to uncover why it was that a man would access these alternative approaches as opposed to going to the traditional mainstream services on offer. The study involved interviews with boys and men who had used the services as well as fieldwork, where the researchers were present at the sessions run by the team to see what was happening at first-hand (White & Cash 2005). There were also interviews with the team members to get their perspective on what was being achieved, or not, and the latest phase of this study is to now seek the main stakeholders' opinions on the service.

BOX 1.1 Key findings from team member interviews

- The team tended not to discuss men's health in terms of disease processes or life expectancy, more in terms of lifestyle and public health issues such as smoking, alcohol and drugs.
- Where health issues were identified as being particularly problematic for men, such as the issue of prostate and testicular cancer, hypertension, diabetes etc., these were from an educational or screening context rather than from a treatment perspective.
- Men do care about their health, whether it be their physical, sexual or emotional health.
- Men are more than willing to discuss issues such as fatherhood, relationship problems and other broader issues as well as their physical health, but men lack the opportunities to discuss these concerns with health professionals because they perceive the health service as a place you go to when you are 'poorly', or because of the social constraints placed on them through being a man.
- The team did recognise that there was a difference between how younger men and older men saw their health and that there is a tendency for men to take the body for granted until age becomes a factor.
- The use of 'incentives' (such as time out of work, free condoms, or special events) was very helpful in getting men and boys to access the services
- The team were able to link the men to other services, either to explain how the systems worked or through direct referral to the general practitioner (GP) etc.
- It is important to be seen as a professional with expert knowledge and to be offering the services that men want.

The interviews with the team gave an insight not only into how they viewed the health of men and what did and didn't work, but also the personal attributes that are required to undertake this form of work and to be successful in outreach work with men (*see* Box 1.1) (this theme is developed in Chapter 14).

From the interviews with the men and from the fieldwork there were findings that supported the views of the team (*see* Box 1.2).

BOX 1.2 Key findings from men

- There was a perception that the GPs were an 'illness service' where you went when 'poorly'.
- The men were reluctant to 'bother the doctor' with what they perceived to be trivial or potentially embarrassing problems.
- A common response was that they would 'go if it was needed' but the tendency was to 'see what it's like tomorrow'.
- Some men seemed to have a lack of confidence in the doctor's ability, with a 'what do they know?' mentality being present.
- The men did not see the GP surgery as a place they felt comfortable taking the kinds of issues that they would talk to the HoM team about.
- There was anxiety in some of the younger men that the GPs were too close to their families, so that there was a strong possibility that parents or others might get to know that they had been to the surgery.
- Health centres don't fit with the way that men like to work – men make more snap decisions. They worry about this ache or pain and when they do decide to do something about it they want to do it there and then, a spontaneity that is rare or difficult to manage at a health centre.
- Health centres tend to close early and not open at the weekend, so there appear to be barriers to the working man in accessing clinics. This is a specific problem for men as they are more likely to be working full time, more likely to be working over 48 hours a week and less likely to have a job that involves flexitime.

The picture that emerged was that by the way in which the team were structuring their services and by their own personal attributes they made it easier for the men to come forward and receive support that they acknowledge they wouldn't have sought if that service wasn't being provided.

A key factor in the work of the HoM team is that they were able to structure their services in a way that overcame some of the difficulties the men were experiencing in using conventional health care. For instance, some of the Asian lads interviewed were very worried that if they spoke to their GP their parents would find out and so they avoided going with anything other than a medical condition that would not cause them problems. With the provision of the anonymity of the Lads' Room they felt safe in discussing issues relating to their sexual health.

The HoM services seemed to provide a safe space that enabled the men to feel more secure in coming forward for a health check and in part this appeared to be a result of the team working on the same wavelength and talking the same language as the men. This required the team to use strategies that made them and their messages sufficiently appealing so that the men were willing to take the risk of exposing their vulnerabilities to these strangers. In part, this was achieved by having the perseverance to be able to keep a service going whilst it developed a reputation within the local male community. It was also through the use of appropriate incentives, for instance handing out free condoms or arranging for the local lads to have weekends away. The team also went into the men's environment, which the men referred to as their 'comfort zone'.

LOCAL CONTEXT

Bradford district covers 141 square miles and has a population of approximately 481,000. The city was built upon the textile industry, which generated significant local wealth and attracted many immigrants from South Asia. Now the mills are mostly gone, as are employment opportunities, leaving a legacy of poverty, disadvantage and poor health. The premature death rate in Bradford as a whole is 6% above the national average. In the most deprived parts of the city the figure is 50% above the national average.

Bradford has a very diverse population from different ethnic backgrounds, including African-Caribbeans, Ukrainians, Poles and Italians, and one of the UK's largest concentrations of South Asians, mostly originating from rural Pakistan. Bradford's Asian community is expected to rise from 60,000 to 160,000 over the next 30 years. These factors give rise to particular health issues which the HoM project set out to address.

PURPOSE AND OBJECTIVES

The purpose of the HoM project was to address men's health inequalities across the Bradford Metropolitan District by providing and coordinating services which:
❭ promoted good health
❭ combated and prevented ill health
❭ were accessible and attractive to men.

Activities within the project were designed with the following core objectives in mind:
❭ to raise awareness of health issues among men by providing accessible services and information to the local male population
❭ to deliver services and information to men through innovative practices away from traditional health settings

❱ to encourage and facilitate health-enhancing activities and to improve health outcomes in the male population

❱ to generate and maintain a two-way flow of communication between providers and users to ensure the continuing relevance and effectiveness of delivery.

The priorities of the project were established by requests for help, information and advice from clients and fellow workers. A questionnaire was used to ascertain more general health needs, and GPs throughout Bradford were surveyed to identify their perceptions of the needs of male patients.

ETHOS

The project set out to be:

❱ *holistic in approach* – addressing the entire spectrum of men's health; physical, emotional and mental

❱ *preventative* – for many men, if not the majority, physical, emotional and mental health issues are interrelated. Often, only physical effects are taken note of, while many problems are exacerbated by ignoring earlier symptoms

❱ *inclusive* – delivery would be sensitive to the particular views and needs of the disparate communities which make up the population of Bradford

❱ *cross-boundary* – not only in the literal sense of working across what were originally four separate PCTs within Bradford District but in providing a presence where health issues are not normally visible, bringing a 'men's health' dimension to the activities of community, voluntary and faith organisations and working with teachers, sports organisers, business owners and youth services.

FUNDING

The first question that many people used to ask was 'How do you get funding to do male health work?' and it must be said that things have changed dramatically over the past five to seven years. When HoM started there were lots of small-scale opportunities to bid for funding to address identified gaps in health delivery to men. The health inequalities men have was a major area of funding, but other angles such as the delivery of services in unique ways (pubs, leisure services, council departments) were all seen as very different five years ago. It shows how far the men's health movement has evolved to see this work as commonplace today in many parts of the country. Funding can be found but it is often from the private and non-statutory sector.

The major turning point for HoM came when we applied for the National Lottery *Healthy Living Centre* scheme. We started with some very grand ideas that could have seen the Men's Health Team touring round Bradford in a bus that had previously been used by the Rolling Stones. Unfortunately, the cost of £700,000 a year in purchase and running costs meant that our claim to rock stardom had to be parked, like the bus! These early dreams were necessary for us to think through the most efficient way to deliver services to men across a district with half a million inhabitants.

The HoM project is as relevant today as it was when we started, but there are many different levers that we now need to pull to keep the funding and goodwill flowing. HoM always had a business-minded approach to everything that we did and the projects that were undertaken by the team could always be marketed both to fellow NHS service providers and the voluntary sector. With the rise of commissioning and provider splits, this business ethos is more relevant than ever. The growing interest in social marketing and social enterprise also gives HoM many opportunities to expand, yet we remain committed to adhering to our original aims of reducing health inequalities, not only between men and women, but between men themselves.

CONCLUSION

Whilst not all areas of the HoM team's work are represented here, due to limitations of space, and while we must acknowledge that some groups of men have yet to be specifically targeted, this book seeks to demonstrate what is possible in tackling the needs of men with regard to their health. It shows that the old adage that men are hard to reach has been replaced with the reality that men are hard to avoid, depending on where you are. If the men will not come to you then it is necessary both to look to where they are and also to look to your own provision of service.

CHAPTER 2

Men's health – what's it all about?

ALAN WHITE

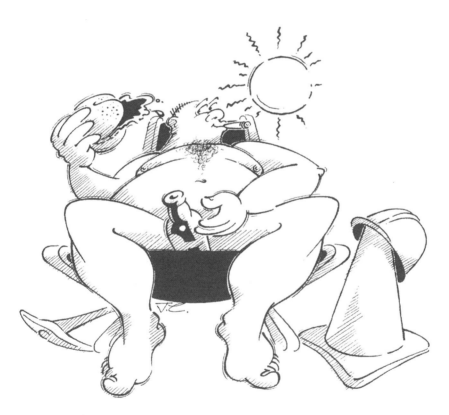

INTRODUCTION

As we learn more about men and their health the more we realise how complex an area it is. We see differences based on age, social class, employment, marital status, ethnicity, sexuality and personal health beliefs and behaviour, all of which can be significantly influenced by life experiences, education and that quirky human trait – free will. To classify all men as the same would therefore be both foolish and completely inaccurate, as there are as many differences between men as there are between men and women. Nevertheless, it seems that there is a need for practitioners to consider how well they are meeting the needs of the men in their care. Each individual man may be different, but when we look at the mortality and morbidity data it does seem that there are issues related to being a man that are significant in explaining why men are so much more at risk of premature death. The conclusion being that something must be happening within every community that makes men so much more vulnerable than women.

In this chapter I will lay out the challenges facing men, from an exploration of the data highlighting the risks men face, to an analysis of men's health beliefs and behaviour, to help explain why the methods outlined in this book seem to strike a chord with so many men and with those who provide health care to them.

Gender duty

There is an added impetus for a book such as this in that in April 2007 new legislation came into force in England and Wales under the *Equality Act 2006* that '. . . require[s] public authorities – as employers or service providers – to actively consider whether they are treating women and men fairly and meeting their different needs' (Department of Trade and Industry 2005 p 14).

This is a major development and one that will have profound implications for many organisations, obliging them to ensure that they have identified the needs of both men and women within their provision and taken steps to meet them. To help implement this legislation, the Equal Opportunities Commission (www.eoc.org.uk) has developed a *Statutory Code of Practice* to accompany the Act, which includes the requirement for all authorities affected by the Act to conduct and publish a gender impact assessment of each 'major' development in policy and services. The code will also be admissible in evidence in any legal action under the *Sex Discrimination Act 1975* or *Equality Act 2006* in criminal or civil proceedings before any court or tribunal. All healthcare providers are now going to have to identify what problems men in their locality face and how their services are meeting their needs.

Defining 'men's health'

Realising the breadth of issues that affect men has meant that defining their health purely in terms of the biological differences with women is insufficient. In their policy document *Getting it Sorted* (2004) the Men's Health Forum (MHF) (England) created a much broader picture that more accurately states the current way of seeing men's health:

> A male health issue is one arising from physiological, psychological, social or environmental factors which have a specific impact on boys or men and/or where particular interventions are required for boys or men in order to achieve

improvements in health and well-being at either the individual or the population level. (MHF 2004)

The challenge that this definition creates is the need for health professionals to consider the broader social environment (rather than be limited to a biomedical perspective), including social care policy, education policy, what is happening in the work environment, what is happening in transport, what is happening in the prison service etc., as well as the personal level.

THE CHALLENGES MEN FACE WITH THEIR HEALTH

There has always been an awareness that men tend to die sooner than women and that men experience cardiovascular problems at an earlier age, accidents are a problem with men's risky lifestyle and there is an increased risk of lung cancer and suicide. These in themselves are sufficient to warrant close attention to how men are targeted, however current studies that have analysed the causes of men's high rate of premature death suggest that men's vulnerability is spread over a far wider range of health problems.

So what are the problems?

Making comparisons with women and their health is not an ideal way of identifying the problems with men and their health, for as we will see there are significant inequalities that exist between men based on socio-economic factors and ethnicity. Comparing men with women also implies that women's health is somehow a standard that men need to reach but this is not the case, as there also exist many serious issues that need to be addressed for women. It has to be acknowledged that it is not possible to fully understand the deficiencies in the health of men unless there is some recognition of difference, especially in areas where one could reasonably expect there to be similarities (i.e. with regard to the non gender-specific illnesses).

Life expectancy

Each year the figures show that both men and women's life expectancy is increasing, with the current figures suggesting that a male child born today should live for 76 years and a female for 82 years. The actual rate of increase is higher for men than for women, which paints a positive picture for health within the country and suggests that men should eventually match women's life expectancy. A closer look at the figures, however, demonstrates that the majority of this increase is coming from improvements in men's health in the highest social class, and that for men in the lowest social class the levels have been predominately the same for a number of years, leading to a widening gap between rich and poor (*see* Figure 2.1). The life expectancy figures given are averages for each social class and in some affluent communities we are finding men living on average into their 80s, whilst in poorer areas the average is down in the 60s. This led the Minister for Public Health to recognise that life expectancy in men is the biggest health inequality issue we face.

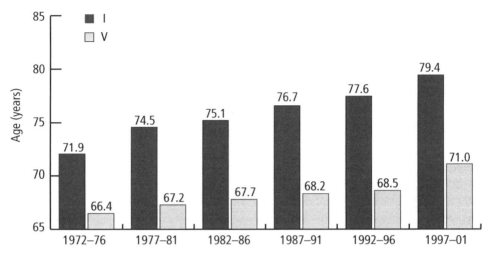

MEN

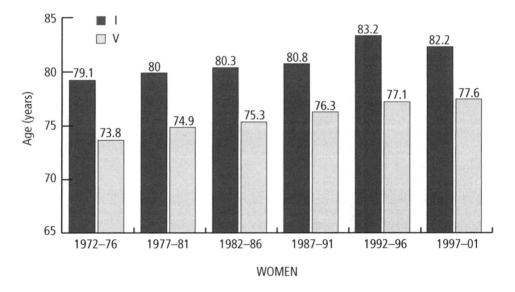

WOMEN

FIGURE 2.1 Relative impact of socio-economic factors on life expectancy.

As part of a study in patterns of mortality in men and women aged 15–44 years (White & Holmes 2006) the ratio of the rate of death across each age group for men and women was calculated, it was found that in the UK young men are twice as likely to die as young women (*see* Figure 2.2) and that throughout the lifespan the proportion of men dying is greater than that of women. Analysis into the patterns of mortality for 15–44 year old men and women gives some insight into why this large difference exists (White & Holmes 2006).

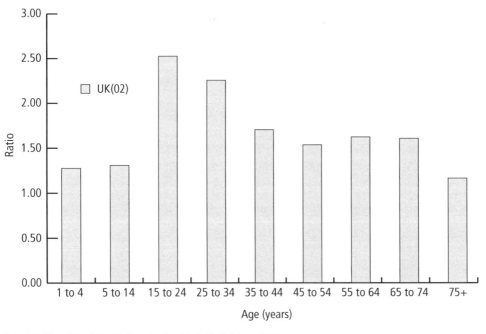

Calculated from World Health Organization Mortality Database 2005

FIGURE 2.2 The ratio between men and women for death from all causes for the UK (2002).

We can see from Figure 2.3 that deaths as a result of accidents and their adverse effects account for the majority of deaths in the 15–34 age bracket, with road traffic accidents accounting for a significant number of those. There are also a substantial number of young men's lives lost to suicide.

When the figures for 35–44 year olds are considered it can be seen that in men that are still classed as 'young' there are a significant number of lives lost from cardiovascular disease (CVD) and cancer. Comparing the figures with those for women there is a similar rise in young womens' deaths from malignant neoplasms, with the majority of these being a result of breast cancer, but the deaths from other causes remain relatively low, such that once the sex specific cancers (breast, cervix, uterus and testis) are removed from the equation men seem to fare badly from all causes of death that should affect men and women equally.

This bears out the findings of a study of the state of men's health across 17 Western European countries (White & Cash 2004), where for all the major causes of death it was only over the age of 75 years that the number of women succumbing outnumbered men.

When the mortality data from the 17 countries was broken down by age and condition it was found that the proportion of men dying was greater in

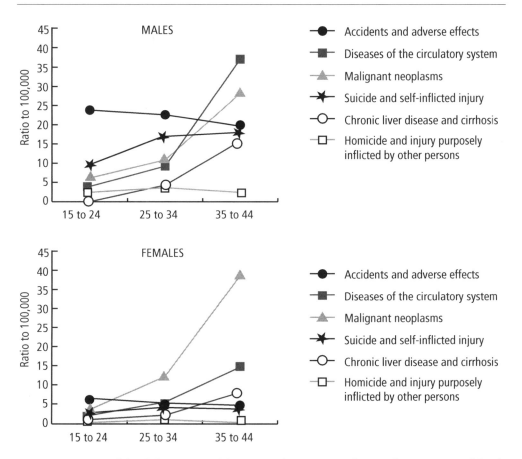

FIGURE 2.3 Rates of death (per 100,000) for men and women, aged 15-44, for six causes of death, United Kingdom, 2002.

the younger age brackets across the majority of causes of death. This suggests that when we are discussing the need for services targeting men we need to be looking beyond the obvious and starting to recognise the breadth of problems which men face.

CONTEXT

To find the reasons why men's health is problematic we need to look at a number of factors. These include whether their biological make-up, the social pressures they are under and, finally, society's expectations of them, put men at risk.

Biophysiological implications of being a male

With every cell having either an XX or an XY genetic base, the biological variations between men and women appear from conception and have fundamental implications for the way we develop and how our bodies work.

There are implications in being biologically born a male, with the American Medical Association recognising the following key differences between males and females:

〉 the sex chromosomes
〉 immune response
〉 symptoms, type, and onset of CVD
〉 response to toxins
〉 brain organisation
〉 the experience of pain

(Wizemann & Pardue 2001).

Whilst these can account for some of the reasons for men's increased susceptibility to develop, and die earlier from, conditions that should affect men and women equally, they do not account for them all, such as the large country by country variations or the effects of socio-economic factors. It can be argued that the most significant issues are most certainly not biological but sociocultural in origin and therefore amenable to change.

Social determinants of health

The World Health Organization (WHO) published a report in 2003 (Wilkinson & Marmot 2003) outlining the ten factors (*see* Box 2.1) from within a society that constitute the social determinants of health.

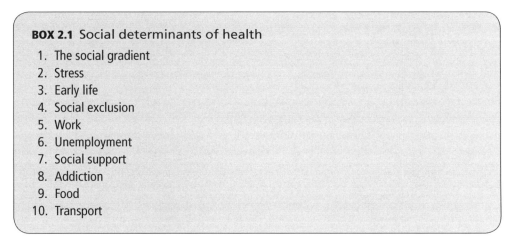

BOX 2.1 Social determinants of health

1. The social gradient
2. Stress
3. Early life
4. Social exclusion
5. Work
6. Unemployment
7. Social support
8. Addiction
9. Food
10. Transport

A brief analysis of these issues with regard to men can highlight why some men find their health so compromised.

The social gradient

Across all the disease states, to a greater or lesser degree, the impact of social inequalities seems to hit men hard. As already mentioned, men from social class five's life expectancy is rising at a much slower rate, and is still three years behind the life expectancy of women in social class five thirty years ago.

Men from different ethnic groups can be seen to have their own particular health challenges with, for instance, African Caribbean men having a threefold greater chance of developing prostate cancer (Kirby & Kirby 2004) and men from South Asia having a four to six times greater chance of developing diabetes (DoH 1999). There are also issues in relation to racism within countries, for instance Royster and colleagues (2006) conducted an epidemiologic study that detailed the experiences of African American men, suggesting that they felt excluded from mainstream healthcare services as a result of their race and economic status and highlighting the concern that different cross sections of society may not be able to derive similar benefits from the same healthcare system. There are additional burdens that men experience, such as the majority of new migrants and asylum seekers being male, with their own difficulties in accessing health services within their new countries.

Stress

Stress is now recognised as being one of the biggest causes of disability at work (and contributes significantly to both the physical and emotional problems of men). There is a growing literature on the emotional development of boys and men and its impact on men's ability to cope with challenges to their mental health (White 2006a). With the tendency of men to shy away from accepting help with emotional problems there is an increased risk of using alcohol and drugs as a way of masking the problem, but further contributing to the difficulties (Brownhill *et al.* 2005). The end result for some is suicide, but along the way can be a catalogue of problems including loss of employment, family breakdown (often as a result of domestic violence) and social isolation.

Early life

Due to the nature of the XY chromosome as compared to the XX chromosome there are a number of problems that boys face from the moment of conception that adversely affect their health. The male embryo is more susceptible to problems of normal gestation and boys are more likely to experience developmental disorders such as specific reading delay, hyperactivity, autism (and related disorders), clumsiness, stammering and Tourette's syndrome, which occur three to four times more in boys (Kraemer 2000). Boys are at least four times more likely to be diagnosed with attention deficit hyperactivity disorder than girls (BUPA 2006). The problems men face later on in their lives are greatly influenced by their ability to gain a good education, but 84% of children excluded from school are boys (Department for Education and Skills (DfES) 2006) and young men are significantly more likely than young women to emerge from the education system with lower levels of qualification.

The socialisation that occurs in this time period also has a significant part to play in how men recognise and deal with their health, which is discussed later.

Social exclusion

Social exclusion can result from poverty, but also from racism, discrimination, stigmatisation, hostility and unemployment (Wilkinson & Marmot 2003); there is also a rising problem of men who are arriving in the UK as asylum seekers or illegal immigrants. Being apart from mainstream society brings with it significant health risks due to the barriers it creates to accessing mainstream health services, education, good housing and support. It is therefore salutatory to note that 73% of adults who go missing are men (Office for National Statistics 2006) and that 90% of people who sleep rough are men (CHAIN 2005).

A major cause of becoming socially excluded is having been through the prison or mental health services. The fact that men make up 94% of the prison population, with 72% of male prisoners suffering from two or more mental disorders (compared with 5% of men in the general population) (Social Exclusion Unit 2003), and that 46% of male psychiatric inpatients (compared with 29% of female patients) are detained and treated compulsorily (MHF 2006) adds considerably to the problems that men face.

Work and unemployment

Ironically both the absence and presence of work can, for some, be a key source of health problems. Within the working environment it is recognised that men are more likely to be involved in potentially dangerous environments, with significantly more men than women suffering work related mortality or disability (White & Cash 2003). The problems that men face are not restricted to hazardous conditions, there are also problems that occur as a result of risk taking within some male cultures, but a principal concern moves the debate away from seeing men as reckless towards recognising that men at work have structural barriers that prevent them seeking appropriate health care.

The new *General Medical Services Contract* means that the majority of men can only access health services if they take time off work. A significant proportion of men work full time, many over 45 hours a week, with only a few having flexitime as an option. Working away from home is now also more common, such that access to the doctor requires having to take a day off work. If it is therefore difficult getting to the doctor when they are ill, it is not surprising that many men find it hard to justify taking a day off work for health screening when they feel that there is actually nothing wrong with them.

For those men who are unemployed there are other challenges. The purpose of work goes beyond monetary gain, bringing a structure to men's lives and a purpose that for many is very hard to replace following redundancy or retirement.

Though an old reference there is still much merit in Johoda's (1979, cited in Freund and McGuire 1991) idea of the 'latency of work', with the actual act of going to work creating:

❭   the imposition of a time structure on the waking day – 'traction'
❭   shared experiences and contacts outside the home

❯ a link for the individual to goals transcending his own purpose – 'sense of purpose' and
❯ the personal standing and identity – 'status'

. . . such that if lost the impact can have wide consequences:
❯ strain in relationships with family and friends
❯ community breakdown in the case of large layoffs (increased crime and other social problems)
❯ loss of self-esteem
❯ problems with structuring time and social identity
❯ where there are additional problems (e.g. psychosis/disability) the experience of unemployment compounds psychological difficulties
❯ increase in suicide, depression, schizophrenia.
(Freund & MacGuire 1991)

Social support

In 2001 a scoping study on men's health (White 2001) was conducted and found four key areas as being central to the discussion on factors influencing men and their health:
❯ access to health services
❯ lack of awareness of their health needs
❯ inability to express their emotions
❯ lack of social networks.

The issue of the lack of social networks related to the difference between men and women with respect to the type of social support available, and that much of men's social capital is built into relationships associated with activities, such as work or sport, as compared with women who have stronger friendships with others willing to help in times of need. This leads to problems for men who through unemployment, disability or the loss of their partner find themselves without any social support. The groups most likely to lack social contacts with relatives, friends and neighbours are divorced or never-married older men, making them more vulnerable to social isolation (Arber *et al.* 2003).

Addiction

There is evidence that the level of smoking in men is decreasing. In 2004/05, 26% of men and 23% of women were cigarette smokers, compared with the early 1970s when around 50% of men and 40% of women smoked. Male smokers smoked more cigarettes a day on average than female smokers. In each year since 1998/99 men smoked on average 15 cigarettes a day compared with 13 for women (Office for National Statistics 2006) but there are still over 17,000 deaths a year as a result of lung cancer and smoking is still a leading cause of cardiac death in men, such that complacency is inappropriate.

Drugs and alcohol, though not causing the same level of premature mortality, still have major implications for men especially as one man in eight is dependent on alcohol, men are three times more likely than women to become alcohol dependent (Office for National Statistics 2001), men are more than twice as likely to use Class A drugs (Roe 2005) and 74% of drug-related deaths occur in men (DrugScope 2006). The increased risk of death is just one aspect of the story, however, with the social and health related consequences on users and their families adding significantly to the burden addiction brings.

Food

The problem of being overweight has tended to be seen as a female issue. Nevertheless, while more women than men are obese there are more overweight men, with the numbers increasing rapidly. It is now estimated that three-quarters of British men will be overweight by 2010 (White & Pettifer 2007).

This rapid increase can be seen to be partially a result of significant changes in society, such as:
> changes in eating patterns
> increasingly sedentary lifestyle
> decline in manual labour
> reduction in walking
> reduced opportunity for exercise
> alcohol consumption
> long working hours.

The relevance of weight to men is that they tend to deposit fat within their abdomen, leading to the apple shape of men, as compared to the pear shape of women whose fat tends to be deposited in their hips and thighs. This visceral fat in men is problematic as it is not an inert substance but has its own endocrine function, with the creation of fat toxins that can lead to the fat related cancers, such as prostate, testis, bowel, liver, kidney, oesophagus and stomach. It also leads to a higher risk of developing hypertension, hyperlipidaemia, and diabetes as a result of the metabolic syndrome. Erectile dysfunction (ED), increased risk of dementia and sleep apnoea are also seen as a consequence of excess weight.

The problem is also compounded by men's relationship with their weight and with food. The social pressure on boys is to be a 'big man', with the muscular body being seen as the ideal. The effect of this is that normal sized boys have been found to see themselves as underweight, as opposed to girls who when a normal weight see themselves as overweight, due to their social conditioning. For instance, in a study of 813 men and women between the ages of 19–39 years, 28–68% of normal weight boys felt they were underweight, while 30–67% of normal weight girls felt they were fat (McCreary & Sadava 2001), so that young women tended to diet to lose weight whereas young men diet to put weight on (McCreary & Sasse 2002).

Transport

The problems relating to transport come in a number of guises, both the health consequences of risk taking in men and boys and the implications of the mode of transport on men's activity levels being problematic.

The consequences of risk taking are seen most strikingly in young men, whose rates of death are significantly higher than women as a result of motor vehicle accidents, both as pedestrians and riders/drivers (White & Holmes 2006). The other side of the health risk is due to the consequences of being behind the wheel, especially in men who are professional drivers such as taxi drivers or lorry drivers, who have been found to be at increased risk of becoming overweight.

Other factors in relation to men's health risks

Though this list seems to be very comprehensive it does not explore why men are at risk, only the outward manifestation of the problem. To look for the cause we need to explore what goes to make up a man and this requires an examination of masculinity.

Masculinity and male socialisation

In a fascinating study in the 1960s, a researcher called Garfinkel (1967) followed the experiences of a man who had a sex change operation and was now entering society as a woman called 'Agnes'. What he found was that just having the body of a male or female did not in itself prepare you for living as a man or woman. Though men and women have a biology and anatomy that distinguishes them physically there are also many other ways in which they are different, to the point that often official or unofficial sanctions are applied to those who do not follow these social rules. Much has been made of these within the popular press, with books such as *Men are from Mars, Women are from Venus* (Gray 1993) being seen as the more extreme end of the published material.

Although in today's society we see much that has encouraged the blurring of boundaries between the sexes, it is possible to see that there are some areas that still link a large majority of men and therefore have relevance to the overall debate about their health. We have a world that has employed methods to segregate men from women, through different expectations of behaviour, clothing, walking, working, playing, drinking and sexual activity, for instance. From birth, studies have shown that boys are treated differently from girls, with colour (blue for a boy), clothes (dresses vs. trousers), language, the way they are handled, play, toys and response to problems ('big boys don't cry') all acting on the developing brain.

Sometimes the policing of these activities is very evident: for instance playground socialisation that dictates what makes a boy a boy is that he is not a girl and therefore does nothing that a girl does (otherwise he will be labelled as a girl or 'gay', Frosh *et al.* 2002). There are also structural pointers that influence how all men see themselves, for instance the use of separate toilets and changing facilities, and it is not that long ago that we had male only pubs, clubs and workplaces. In addition, we are bombarded with media messages as to how men should and should not perform and how they should look.

All these combine to create an image of what boys and girls can expect from, and their role in, the world they inhabit and, whether men adhere to them or not, they are so pervasive that it is impossible for them not to have left an imprint. All men, no matter what their circumstances, cannot escape the fact that they have been subject to a socialisation process that will have influenced how they see themselves against a 'model' of masculinity and the message that is being pushed fits in well with the idea of hegemonic, or dominant, masculinity put forward by Connell (1995) and Courtenay (2000):

> In exhibiting or enacting hegemonic ideals with health behaviours, men reinforce strongly held cultural beliefs that men are more powerful and less vulnerable than women; that men's bodies are structurally more efficient than and superior to women's bodies; that asking for help and caring for one's health are feminine; and that the most powerful men among men are those for whom health and safety are irrelevant. (Courtenay 2000)

This leaves the individual man with a problem, however. This is a model that does not reflect how the majority of men think or feel, but each and every man knows that this is the expectation of them and is how they should think and behave. It is acknowledged that very few men 'rise' to this stereotypical image, with both groups and individuals standing outside this expectation.

Connell (1995) makes reference to other forms of masculinity:

❭ marginalised – e.g. as a result of ethnicity
❭ complicit – relating to men who do not perform hegemonic masculinity in its purest form, but are able to enjoy the patriarchal dividend that has been created
❭ subordinate masculinities – as experienced by men who are homosexual.

This reinforces the notion that all men, from whatever background and personal philosophy on life, are still at some level aware of a social expectation about how they should perform. They may decide not to follow that 'life way', but the messages they receive will make them aware that there is a model that they are being referenced against.

This constant feeding of messages pushing men to be independent, powerful and proud, with inner strength, competitiveness, achievement at work, success, self-control and physical strength added to a feeling of invincibility (Newman 1997) does little to help men to manage their health. Problems with your health imply weakness, vulnerability and the need for others' help. Of specific concern within this chapter is the question of what this socialisation process does for male help-seeking behaviour.

MEN'S USAGE OF HEALTH SERVICES

It is widely recognised that men don't access family doctors to the same extent as women. Indeed they are not frequent attenders of the majority of services related to health; high street pharmacies are predominately accessed by women and men are less likely to have regular dental checks, eye checks or to access health screening.

In part, this can be linked to the lack of formalised health screening for men and also the fact that for many men their health remains static, without the need to access health services for contraception or antenatal care. Men's bodies are relatively unchanging, with none of the hormonal or physical changes associated with monthly menstruation experienced by women, and this affects men's aware-ness of their bodies. Saltonstall (1993) notes that men tend to take their bodies for granted, with an expectation that it will perform what is expected of it.

The problems that men do encounter with their health, especially in their formative years, tend to be transient, i.e. as a result of infection, over-exertion or accident, or self-induced (alcohol related) and, as such, the typical management strategy is to ignore it and it will go away.

This is compounded for many men by limitations in their ability to access health services, with men at work being a specific example of how structural issues remove from men options in accessing healthcare services.

A further component in the picture as to why men don't use heath services was identified by Davidson & Arber (2003) who found two key categories of non-users of medical services:

❭ *sceptics:* 'Most of them are a waste of time'; 'I don't like doctors, I keep as far away from the place . . . it's not an exact science'; 'meteorology and medicine were about as accurate as each other', 'rather go to a veterinary surgeon than a doctor'

❭ *stoics:* 'I don't give in. Even if I felt awful, I wouldn't tell anyone'; 'You've just got to get through it.'

Lloyd and Forrest's (2001) review of services for young men found a further set of issues when considering if young men would access health services. They found that they would respond when:

❭ they were desperate
❭ access was easy or easier
❭ identity was involved – culture, community base and common experience of racism were often significant factors
❭ they had to be there, i.e. young offenders/school based projects.

The problem with the delay in seeking help is that it results in reduced treatment options available to the physician and in increased risk of unnecessary disability or premature death (White & Banks 2004).

If the data is explored as to men's actual usage of services by age (*see* Figure 2.4) we can see that boys and girls appear to access the services in about equal numbers, but as the teenage years move into early adulthood the difference broadens with increasing age. Nevertheless the gap then narrows again until men exceed women's usage for the over-75 year olds.

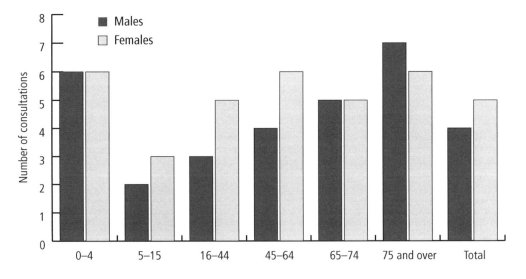

FIGURE 2.4 Consultations per year for men and women, by age.

When socio-economic influences are brought into the equation (*see* Figure 2.5) we can see that another picture emerges, where for men there are marked differences based on whether they are in blue collar work or professional workers. For women there are very few differences based upon socio-economic status, only those based on age. The increased use of health services by men from lower socio-economic groups implies both a greater degree of illness and the need for official sanction for their health status.

Current research and literature reviews pertaining to men and help-seeking behaviour suggest that this is a key factor affecting men's overall health (Galdas *et al.* 2005; O'Brien *et al.* 2005). Male socialisation, which militates against showing vulnerability and an inability to cope, coupled with problems in accessing healthcare services, creates significant problems for men in knowing when and how to access appropriate assistance. In a scoping study on men's health (White 2001) the issue of men accessing healthcare services was a principal cause for concern, with the survey respondents noting the following as key factors in men's difficulties with gaining appropriate health support:

》 a lack of understanding of the processes of making appointments and negotiating with female receptionists
》 inappropriate office opening times, which tend to coincide and conflict with work commitments
》 an unwillingness to wait for appointments

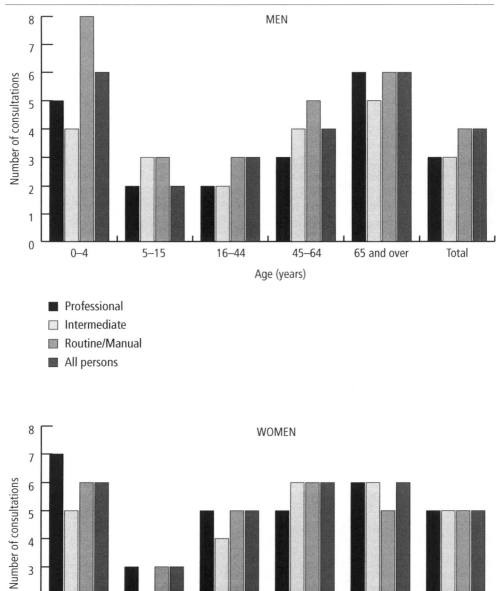

www.statistics.gov.uk/STATBASE/ssdataset.asp?vlnk=5435 (accessed Jan 2004)

FIGURE 2.5 GP consultations per year by age and socio-economic status.

> a feeling that the service is primarily for women and children, and that sitting in the waiting room is uncomfortable for them
> the name 'health centre' has been identified as problematic
> the negative response many men feel they get when presenting with difficulties that are not quickly dealt with
> a lack of trust in the healthcare system, mainly around the issue of confidentiality, especially within the gay community and regarding disclosure of HIV status
> great fears relating to shame if their concerns are judged to be of little consequence, or having to admit to another person that they may have a problem, namely one that they can't solve themselves
> lacking the vocabulary they feel is necessary to discuss issues of a sensitive nature, with the result that it is easier to go to the doctor with a non-embarrassing physical illness than when depressed or faced with the symptoms of, for example, colorectal cancer or ED.

What is being recognised is that the traditional GP services are excellent in providing a diagnostic and treatment service, but there appears to be a problem for men in both recognising their health needs and being aware of how to use the current health service to gain maximum effect. For instance, the man with hypertension will gain appropriate care, but only if he knows that he has a problem and that it necessitates having his blood pressure (BP) checked, or the man with emotional difficulties can receive referral for cognitive behavioural therapy, but only if he presents with the problem.

This recognition of the limited success that conventional services were having on targeting men successfully was the impetus for the Bradford team to set up their dedicated services for men.

CHAPTER 3

Introduction to health promotion
RUTH CROSS

INTRODUCTION
This chapter aims to:

⟩ introduce the reader to the concept of health promotion
⟩ clarify commonly used terms
⟩ give a brief history of the development of health promotion
⟩ explore key concepts within health promotion i.e. principles and values, ways of working, approaches to health promotion and settings for promoting health
⟩ explore what works in promoting men's health.

WHAT IS HEALTH PROMOTION?
'Health promotion' is not easy to define. There are difficulties with defining what 'health' is in the first the place, so determining what we mean by health promotion depends on what we mean by health. What exactly are we promoting? The concept of health is debated and contested. It has even been described as 'nebulous' (Tones *et al.* 1994). The meaning of health to individuals and collective groups is subjective and influenced by a wide range of factors. These include culture, socio-economic factors and, of course, gender. What health means to one person will not necessarily be representative of what health means to another. Health can be viewed as a positive state (in terms of wellbeing or even happiness), a negative state (as absence of disease or disability), a resource for living and adapting effectively to life's circumstances or quality of life, to name a few stances. The advantage of this is that, since health means so many different things to different people, there are many different ways to promote health. If health is viewed as having several different dimensions, a great many activities

and ways of working can promote health – although some might be more obvious than others. Of course, this can prove challenging when trying to promote health in practice.

Health experience and concepts of health vary considerably between, and within, groups. It is no different with men. Men's health experience varies, for example, from one socio-economic group or community to another (White 2006b) and so do men's concepts of health. In the case of men, research shows that ideas about 'masculinity' are closely aligned with ideas about health and also with health-related behaviour (De Visser & Smith 2006). Research also shows that, with regard to health, men engage in riskier behaviours and hold riskier beliefs than women (Courtney *et al.* 2002).

Health promotion, as defined by the WHO agenda, operates using a holistic view of health, recognising that health is a complex concept. Health is viewed in a positive rather than negative light – as something worth promoting. Health promotion therefore places a high value on health and wellbeing. Health promotion may be defined or described in two ways: firstly as a way of working, and secondly as a set of guiding principles and values underpinning ways of working.

Health promotion illustrates a move away from purely focussing on a biomedical view of health towards an understanding that health is also socially constructed. Historically, the biomedical model of health has focussed on a negative, mechanistic view of health rooted in scientific, objective thought. Emphasis has been on diagnosis, treatment and cure of disease. This has resulted in a tendency to place responsibility for health with the individual at the expense of considering wider influences on health experience. Whilst the importance of lifestyle choices cannot be ignored, this has occurred at the expense of appreciating the wider arena in which 'health' is played out and experienced – the socio-economic, political and environmental context.

Health promotion seeks to view health in a much more holistic way, taking into account wider determinants and factors influencing health. Issues such as tackling inequalities in health are at the centre of health promoting practice. Inequalities in health are evident in a wide range of ways from a macro or global scale to more local or micro examples. Men are not immune from inequalities in health and the evidence that they lag behind women in many ways in terms of health experience is overwhelming. For example, in a pan-European study looking at the state of men's health across 17 European countries carried out by White and Cash (2003) the number of male deaths was around twice the number of female deaths from age 1 year to age 74 years.

The argument for promoting health is that there are many diseases of our time in western societies that are preventable. The biggest threats to men's health at the current time are chronic diseases often associated with lifestyle choices and behaviour. These are CVDs such as coronary heart disease and stroke, diabetes and cancers, accidents, unintentional injury and suicide, kidney, liver and respiratory diseases. Most of these kill more men than women when you compare age of death. This means that men, on average, live shorter lives than women. Herein lies the argument for promoting men's health. Since the major diseases of the time in the UK context are, in part, preventable, significant risk reduction for the individual can be achieved by reducing, increasing or moderating certain behaviours. These behaviours include tobacco use, alcohol use, exercise uptake, dietary choices, risk taking and sexual behaviour. It is well accepted that generally a variation in risk behaviours and risk exposure exists between men and women, with men demonstrating higher risk in both areas. This has implications for health promotion for men.

There is a place for both individual and structural approaches to promoting health to enable positive sustainable changes to effect health. However, the focus so far has been very much on the individual rather than the wider factors impacting on health that were presented earlier. Nonetheless, it is not all about persuading men to change their behaviour, although this is an important part of promoting men's health. It is also about tackling the societal and structural factors that impact on men's lives and enabling sustainable change through providing supportive environments. This calls for multidisciplinary and multi-sectoral ways of working and includes measures such as working with society in general, for example, to change attitudes and challenge norms and values. An example is the link that has been found between masculinity, i.e. ideas of men having to be 'macho', and the negative impact that this has on men's health. It also means working to influence policy and tackling the root causes of health inequalities, such as poverty, disadvantage and deprivation which affect men as well as women and children.

A BRIEF HISTORY OF HEALTH PROMOTION: THE WHO'S AGENDA – FROM ALMA ATA TO BANGKOK

The WHO (1986) defines health promotion as 'the process of enabling people to increase control over, and to improve, their health'. The definition goes on to state that 'to reach a state of complete physical, mental and social well-being, an individual or group must be able to identify and to realise aspirations, to satisfy needs, and change or cope with the environment'. Health is therefore seen as a resource for everyday life, not the objective of living. Health is a positive concept emphasising social and personal resources, as well as physical capabilities. Therefore, health promotion is not just the responsibility of the health sector, but goes beyond healthy lifestyles to wellbeing, reinforcing the holistic nature of health.

The WHO has, in many ways, been at the forefront of developments in health promotion for the last few decades. In 1977 the *Alma Ata Declaration* resulted from the meeting of the WHO at the World Health Assembly. An ambitious goal was declared – 'Health for all by the year 2000'. The means of achieving this goal was through primary health care. Although positive advances in health have been made, this goal has not been achieved. The focus of the declaration was on prevention and it put key issues onto the health agenda such as social justice, addressing inequalities and governmental responsibility.

The *Ottawa Charter* on health promotion (1986) resulted from the first international conference on health promotion held by the WHO in Ottawa, Canada. The charter laid out the following areas for action for promoting health:

) building healthy public policy
) creating supportive environments
) strengthening community action
) developing personal skills
) reorienting health services.

This was to be achieved by three strategic ways of working – advocacy, enabling and mediation.

The second international conference on health promotion was held in 1988 in Adelaide, Australia. It focussed on healthy public policy and advocated the creation of supportive environments and alliances for health. The third was held in Sundsvall, Sweden in 1991 and resulted in the *Sundsvall Statement on Supportive Environments for Health*, building on previous developments. In 1997 the fourth international health promotion conference, held in Jakarta, reinforced health as a basic human right, identified settings as key to promoting health and set out the following priorities for health promotion in the 21st century:

) promote social responsibility for health
) increase investments for health development
) consolidate and expand partnerships for health
) increase community capacity and empower the individual
) secure an infrastructure for health promotion.

The fifth international conference on health promotion, held in Mexico in 2000, built on previous strategic developments highlighting the need to invest in health and create an infrastructure for health promotion to reduce inequity. The sixth was held in Bangkok in 2005 and the resulting *Bangkok Charter* emphasised the need to address determinants of health.

Themes running through the WHO agenda for health promotion which can be seen as a basis for ways of working include health as a basic human right, health as a resource for living, addressing inequalities and inequities, social justice, empowerment, influencing policy for health, working in partnerships and creating supportive environments.

WAYS OF WORKING

Health promotion is often referred to as an umbrella term (Tones & Green 2004), acknowledging that there are numerous ways of working. The range of interventions and processes that may be referred to as promoting health is therefore wide reaching. For example, activities intended to promote men's health may be as diverse as *Men's Health Week* (run by the Men's Health Forum), creation of websites, mobile health screening etc.

Health promotion may be broadly divided into two ways of working – a top-down approach or a bottom-up approach. The top-down approach tends to be expert led, where the health needs of a community are defined and determined by 'outsiders' who might be healthcare professionals, health experts or other agents. An example, in promoting men's health, of a top-down approach is screening for prostate cancer. Bottom-up approaches on the other hand mean that the 'insiders', i.e. the community themselves, determine what their health needs are and how to go about addressing them. An example in promoting men's health using a bottom-up approach is the focus of *Men's Health Week 2006* on emotional wellbeing – a response to findings from surveying men about their mental health. Both ways of working have their place in promoting men's health and often a combination of the two is used in practice.

APPROACHES TO HEALTH PROMOTION

In addition to the two approaches already discussed much of current health promotion literature refers to several other approaches within health promotion. Naidoo and Wills (2000) identify five approaches which are useful in describing the way that health promoters work. These are the 1) medical approach, 2) the behaviour change approach, 3) the educational approach, 4) the empowerment approach and 5) the social change approach (sometimes also referred to as the socio-environmental approach). Each approach has a different focus, evident from the description of the approach itself.

The medical approach would refer to activities directed at reducing death rates or early deaths and minimising ill health by targeting certain groups or populations. The medical approach is also concerned with prevention. There are commonly three levels of prevention defined in the wider health promotion literature – primary prevention, secondary prevention and tertiary prevention. Primary prevention focusses on preventing ill health occurring with the well individual and involves action to keep the healthy person healthy. This might include for example, encouraging healthy lifestyle choices, uptake of immunisation etc. Secondary prevention focusses on identifying illness or disease in its very early stages through means such as screening. Tertiary prevention focusses on preventing the progression of an illness, the aim being to return to a state of 'health' or minimise residual disability. An example of primary prevention would be encouraging young men to drink less than the government's recommended number of alcohol units per week, an example of secondary prevention would be encouraging prostate cancer screening at early onset of associated symptoms, and an example of tertiary prevention would be maintaining blood sugars within an acceptable range for a man with diabetes.

The behaviour change approach focusses on individual behaviours – reducing, eliminating, commencing or increasing certain behaviours dependent on the nature of the behaviour in question and whether it impacts negatively or positively on health. The educational approach aims to provide knowledge and information so that people can develop skills and make informed choices about their health and their health behaviour (Naidoo & Wills 2000). The empowerment approach is key to promoting health and at the forefront of the WHO agenda as previously identified. It is about increasing people's power and control over their lives to make a difference to their health experience. Empowerment may occur at an individual or community level. An example of working in a more empowering way with communities is the community development approach. The social change approach is concerned with addressing the wider environment impacting on health, taking into account factors such as economics, environment and politics.

Each approach to promoting health has its opportunities and challenges and operates within its own set of values and principles. Health promotion interventions do not often use these approaches exclusively, so more than one approach may be evident in any given programme or intervention.

SETTINGS FOR PROMOTING MEN'S HEALTH

The settings approach to health promotion has its roots in the WHO's agenda dating from the Ottawa Charter. Arguably, all settings are ones in which health maybe promoted or demoted, whether these settings are public or private in nature. Commonly identified settings for health promotion include, for example, schools, hospitals, the workplace, the home and neighbourhoods. Settings may be physical, social or, in an age of increasing technological advances and the World Wide Web, even virtual. Settings more specific to promoting the health of men may be seen to be pubs, barber shops or prisons, for example – basically anywhere where men are in the majority. This is demonstrated by the issues and examples discussed in this book. The Men's Health Forum website (www. menshealthforum.org.uk) gives good examples of recent and current projects in men's health promotion in a range of different settings such as prisons, colleges, healthy living centres, pubs etc.

The argument for pursuing men in less 'traditional' settings for promoting health is that men are 'hard to reach', in terms of health, for many reasons. Research shows, for example, that men are reluctant to seek help, they delay seeking help, and are less likely to see a doctor if they feel ill or to report symptoms of ill health once they occur. If the men won't come to the health services, the health services must go to the men. The sort of questions to ask therefore, in terms of settings for promoting men's health, are 'where are men?' and 'where do men go?'. The answers vary – workplaces, pubs and bars are good examples. A distinction may be made between health promotion *in* a setting (settings providing access to men, for example) and a settings *approach* whereby all aspects of a specific setting contribute to promoting health.

MEN AS A TARGET GROUP

A great deal of health promotion intervention is targeted at certain sectors of the general population. The degree to which this is appropriate will depend on the aims of the specific intervention and also the nature of the health issue in hand. Initiatives and interventions to promote men's health are mostly aimed at men, although this is not necessarily the case (for example, research shows that women are often 'gatekeepers' for men's health, particularly with regards to issues such as diet, help seeking etc.). Within the broader target group of 'men' certain men may also be targeted, such as younger men, older men, gay men, men at university, men in manual employment etc.

THE CHALLENGE OF PROMOTING MEN'S HEALTH

It is quite often a challenge to prove what works in promoting health. This is for a variety of reasons. Many a theoretical debate has taken place in the discipline as to what constitutes evidence of success. Evidence may be statistical or anecdotal. Difficulties in measuring success result from issues such as defining key terms, the subjective nature of health and the long-term approach of most interventions in health promotion – changes and results may not be seen for many years. Examples from research indicate that certain ways of working to promote men's health are more appropriate, acceptable and effective, such as workplace health promotion campaigns.

It is important for those working to positively influence men's health that health promotion interventions result from looking at the determinants of men's health and address these in some way. This will often include consideration of environmental and structural influences as well as influences on behaviour itself. Since men are more exposed to behavioural risk, for example, understanding *why* this is the case will enable health promotion interventions to be planned more appropriately and with greater effect, taking into consideration such things as cultural and social beliefs and subsequent influences on masculinity.

CONCLUSION

What should be evident from this chapter is that health promotion encompasses a range of activities and that lots of people, in a variety of diverse roles, 'do' health promotion or actually 'promote health' – not just healthcare professionals themselves but a wide range of people working in a wide range of roles, from policy makers to teachers to community workers. Concepts of health and health promotion are broad and diverse, and therefore promoting health encompasses many ways of working.

PART TWO

CHAPTER 4

Health MOTs

PETE WESTWOOD AND ANDREW HARRISON

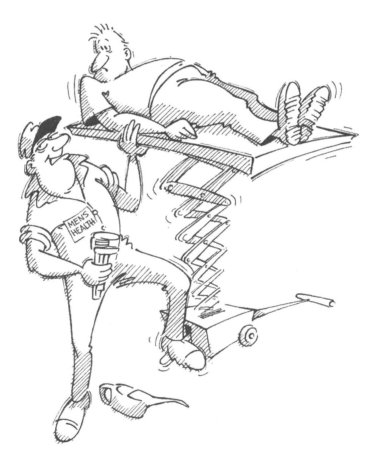

INTRODUCTION

Men like gadgets. This is highlighted by the amount of care and attention that they bestow on their bicycles, motorbikes and cars. Regular maintenance and checks (tyre pressure, oil and water) are carried out, engine specifications are known and if problems occur, men will put safety first and sort them out.

So, why do men not look after their most precious possessions – their bodies? Ask a man if he knows his BP reading and he probably won't, ask him his waist size and he will lie, ask him how he feels . . . well don't even go there.

In an effort to address this imbalance, health MOTs have been designed to provide a health check in a manner with which many men can identify. It is an opportunity to have a detailed review of their current health, to receive advice on health matters and to discuss any aspect of their health and wellbeing. It is an idea that has developed locally and nationally, culminating in the recent health White Paper (2006), which responded to the growing expressed desire of the population that they don't want to be 'nannied' or told what to do, but they do want more information, advice and support.

Health MOTs, or simple health checks, are nothing new. They come in different formats and are available in numerous locations, such as workplaces, leisure centres and GP surgeries.

The HoM team developed and expanded DeVille-Almond's (2002) approach, which targeted the 'at risk' and 'hard to reach' groups of men.

WHERE DO I OFFER HEALTH MOTS?

Answer – wherever men are. HoM MOTs have been delivered in numerous locations:

 ❯ workplaces (small and large multinational companies with a predominantly male workforce)
 ❯ locations within the community such as: mosques, community centres, pubs, barbers' shops and saunas
 ❯ at specific events (for example, working in partnership with Age Concern to target men aged over 50) and on an ad hoc basis if appropriate.

With some exceptions, men will rarely take the initiative or the time to venture into a *Well Man* clinic for a health check, and so the aim is to venture outside the usual National Health Service (NHS) boundaries and work wherever men are.

HOW DO I GET 'IN'?

 ❯ Make effective use of established contacts. For example, by working with a health promotion colleague within Bradford council, we had an opportunity to access over 300 street cleaners and refuse collectors.
 ❯ Think about ways to get free publicity. The success of HoM's early work generated interest in local business magazines and later in more mainstream media sources – namely radio and local newspapers.
 ❯ Opportunistic cold calling. Sometimes this can be very successful (e.g. with setting up HoM MOTs in a barber shop used by people from South Asia), and sometimes not. Often we found that the NHS logo sold itself as people trusted the service.

⟩ By word of mouth. This was so effective for us that we're now more selective in deciding which organisations to work in, e.g. companies without occupational health departments. Let's remember, however, that unhealthy men are not selective as to which companies they work for.

⟩ Through committed and interested individuals, for instance, union representatives, health and safety officers, occupational health nurses and community leaders.

WHAT DOES AN MOT CONSIST OF?

A typical MOT will take at least 30–45 minutes. Think of that – a man investing an unhurried, uninterrupted half an hour of his time to consider and talk about his health! It will involve some clinical measurements, some questioning on lifestyle and knowledge of pertinent health issues and then a review of the health status of the individual man based on all of this information. It is very much a participative exercise and should not be threatening or unduly confrontational in nature. While there is often a lot of information to pass on, it is also important that the health professional is a good listener, in order to ensure maximum potential for the client to discuss the issues that matter to him:

⟩ **Measurements** These usually include BP, pulse, height and weight (for body mass index (BMI)), waist measurement, blood cholesterol, blood glucose and carbon monoxide (CO) if a smoker.

⟩ **Lifestyle review** This may include questioning regarding smoking, alcohol, eating and exercise.

⟩ **Discussion** Including issues such as family history of illness, current medications, emotional wellbeing, sexual health, male-specific illnesses such as prostate and testicular cancer and general health topics.

WHAT ARE THE BENEFITS TO THE CLIENT?

Men derive different benefits from the MOT session, but the men may be summarised as follows:

⟩ *The worried well* These men sometimes come along for reassurance that everything is alright. They may not have reviewed their health with a nurse or doctor for many years and wish to 'have a bit of a check up'. All may be in order but there is merit in a measure of positive feedback. Clearly, these are not the most productive clients in terms of the use of time and resources, but nor should they be seen as unimportant.

⟩ *Time to think again* These men have benefited from the balanced review of their health and have come to realise that maybe it is time to make some changes. Possibly they need to modify their drinking habits, or address their increasing waist measurements. Maybe they need to think more deeply about how they might incorporate physical exercise into their work, social and family lives. The health worker may assist in working through these issues but may equally be just the catalyst for change.

❭ *Needs some attention* These men discover that one or more of their clinical measurements is out of the normal range according to the relevant clinical standards. They may be hypertensive or have high cholesterol readings. They may require referral to another health professional for review, again in accordance with agreed clinical and referral protocols.

❭ *Get help now!* Occasionally we find men who require urgent referral to a specialist medical service. An MOT can save a life! (*see* Elliott 2005)

☆ HANDY HINT

The client may wish to speak in depth about a single issue that's been worrying him. This is often a very personal issue that he has hitherto found himself unable to raise with anyone, e.g. marriage problems, stress, ED or difficulties in finding a healthy work/home life balance.

WHAT ARE THE BENEFITS TO EMPLOYERS?

There is now an increasing awareness of the potential short-term and long-term benefits of health promotion and a more proactive approach in relation to personal health care. Statistics abound regarding the rate of work-related ill health and the number of working days lost due to ill health. It is clearly to the advantage of employer and employee alike to ensure that health is a priority.

Additionally, there is often an increased feeling of goodwill between employers and employees when it is clear that 'management' are taking an interest in the health and wellbeing of the workforce.

WHAT ELSE DO I NEED TO KNOW?

Be sure to act within the clinical guidelines of the employing organisation. This might mean that you need to meet with the relevant specialist services and clinical leads. There might even be some 'professional protectionism'!

Consider how you might evaluate the effectiveness of your MOT work. Basic data including the number of clients and the number that are referred on to specialist services are easy to collate. Less easy is the *effect* of your work. With the HoM MOTs it was necessary to hand over responsibility to the individual client to contact his GP or other health professional in the event of a clinical problem. Although we are confident that a high proportion of clients *did* indeed make contact, it is difficult to prove this and provide meaningful statistics.

We've had no feedback from GPs regarding any referrals we have made to them. A possible solution to this is to share information electronically by contributing to the GPs' own information database. This has thus far been resisted on the grounds of confidentiality.

The MOT package when supplied to large companies has often created a useful referral pathway to weight management and smoking cessation groups led by our team within the workplace. This face to face contact is crucial to the process by which men take that step from thinking about their health to actually doing something about it. The subsequent groups are particularly useful in that they provide hard data of the effectiveness of the health activity in the workplace.

☆ HANDY HINT

The HoM MOTs have evolved and adapted since our first ventures into this area. Over time, changes have been made both to the format and style of the sessions. This process has involved much debate as the team have reflected and grappled with various dilemmas.

The contact person in a workplace or community venue is often the factor which determines the success of the MOT programme – certainly in terms of the numbers of 'takers' but also in the quality of the individual consultations. If the contact person is very knowledgeable about the workforce he/she will be able to effectively draw in the men. He/she may also be able to target the men who are most in need of the service. If he/she is trusted, then it is more likely that the service will be trusted. Are the communication systems effective? Is it simply a case of putting up a few posters and leaving it at that? Or does he/she actively seek out the men who will fill the appointments, take time to organise the event, book rooms and plan appointment times?

Who are you trying to target? Are you satisfied to just get any men to access your service or are you targeting the over 50s, the manual or the blue collar workers? You may want to be specific as to whom you want to access the service and plan how you're going to make sure that this will happen.

☒ WARNING

This quote is from a refuse collector who accessed our MOT service. Just when we thought we were doing well, it brought us back to earth, highlighting the difficulties in engaging with men in the workplace: 'There are some right specimens out there in the yard, but they are **too scared** to come in and see you'.

Who will deliver this work? Will you provide it in-house or will you pull in workers from other organisations. What are the cost implications of this? Are the health professionals adequately experienced and comfortable in promoting men's health? Do they have adequate local knowledge of the services to which men may be signposted? Are there supervision issues regarding untrained or trained nursing staff? Is the organisation that you are working with expecting a service provided by suitably experienced trained nurses?

While all that is really required of the host organisation is a private room with a table and two chairs, are you sure that the working environment will be satisfactory? Is there a break built into the MOT programme and access to a kitchen to make a cup of tea? If not, don't forget your flask and sandwiches. Is there an induction process you are required to attend before you can work on-site?

SUMMARY

Aims	MOTs have been designed to provide a health check in a manner that many men can identify with.
	They are an opportunity for men to have a detailed review of their current health, to receive advice on health matters and to discuss any aspect of their health and wellbeing.
Where do I offer health MOTs?	Men will rarely take the initiative or the time to venture into a *Well Man* clinic for health checks.
	The aim is to venture outside of the usual NHS boundaries and work wherever men are, e.g.
	workplaces, mosques, community centres, pubs, barbers' shops, saunas and at specific events.
How do I get 'in'?	Make effective use of established contacts.
	Opportunistic cold calling.
	Think about ways to get free publicity.
	By word of mouth.
What does an MOT consist of?	A typical MOT will take at least 30–45 minutes, including:
	measurements
	lifestyle review
	discussion
What are the benefits to the client?	*The worried well* These men sometimes come along for some reassurance that everything is alright.
	Time to think again These men have benefited from the balanced review of their health and have come to realise that maybe it is time to make some changes.
	Needs some attention These men discover that one or more of their clinical measurements is out of the normal range.
	Get help now! Occasionally we find men who require urgent referral to a specialist medical service.

What are the benefits to the employer?	Statistics abound regarding the number of working days lost due to ill health.
	There is often an increased feeling of goodwill between employers and employees when it is clear that 'management' are taking an interest in the health and wellbeing of the workforce.
What else do I need to know?	Think about who you're specifically targeting, who will deliver the sessions and whether the work environment offers a suitable place in which to conduct them.
	Consider how you might evaluate the effectiveness of your MOT work.
	The MOT package supplied to a large company has often created a useful referral pathway to weight management and smoking cessation groups led by our team within the workplace.
	The contact person in a workplace or community venue is often the factor which determines the success of the MOT programme.
	Be sure to act within the clinical guidelines of the employing organisation.

CHAPTER 5

Sexual health outreach work

NICK DAVY

INTRODUCTION

This chapter focusses on sexual health promotion in primary care. It would seem appropriate to begin this chapter with a definition of sexual health.

> Sexual health is an important part of physical and mental health. It is a key part of our identity as human beings together with the fundamental human rights to privacy, a family life and living free from discrimination. Essential elements of good sexual health are equitable relationships and sexual fulfilment with access to information and services to avoid the risk of unintended pregnancy, illness or disease. (National Strategy for Sexual Health and HIV 2001)

If you are working in sexual health promotion with young people, however, the above definition might be a little wordy. A 'young people friendly' definition could be:

> Sexual health is an important part of your overall health; it is part of who you are. It includes avoiding sexually transmitted infections and unintended pregnancy, and allowing you sexual expression and enjoyment without exploitation, oppression and abuse.

Here are some key facts.
❱ Research suggests that sexual risk-taking behaviour is increasing across the population.
❱ Chlamydia is the most common sexually transmitted infection. In a survey, awareness of chlamydia as a sexually transmitted infection (STI) declined with

age, especially among men, and only half of men knew that it is easily treated with antibiotics (DoH 2003a).

❭ Delays in detection and access to treatment lead to more people being infected with STIs and the development of complications.

❭ Nearly a quarter of all pregnancies in England and Wales end in abortion.

❭ If a condom was used for every act of unprotected sex with the risk of an unplanned pregnancy or of transfer of an STI, there would be an immediate impact on the STI rate, and significantly fewer unplanned pregnancies and therefore a reduction in abortion.

❭ In a single act of unprotected sex with an infected partner, teenagers have:
   – A 30% chance of getting genital herpes
   – A 50% chance of contracting gonorrhoea.

(Teenage Pregnancy Unit 1999)

With all of the above, it is easy to see why sexual health promotion is so important, for men as well as women. Concordance in condom use is central to the prevention of both pregnancy and the spread of STIs. To help achieve this, it is not enough to provide barrier contraception but we must raise awareness and educate wherever possible.

☞ INFO

The UK has the highest teenage pregnancy rate in Europe (Health Development Agency (HDA) 2003) and an alarmingly high level of STIs, particularly among young people (Health Protection Agency (HPA)2005).

The DoH has said that tackling the rise in STIs is a government priority and has invested an extra £300m in sexual health, as outlined in the *Choosing Health* White Paper (2004b). This includes £40m invested for upgrading contraceptive services. To enable this money to be well spent it is imperative that services work together in partnership and ensure that sexual health plays a key role in local delivery plans aimed specifically at men.

The Independent Advisory Group (IAG) on Sexual Health and HIV (2005) states:

> the IAG wholeheartedly supports the Government in its drive to improve and modernise services and feels it is vital to keep [genito-urinary medicine (GUM)], contraceptive services, and the provision of sexual health services overall, at the forefront of policy initiatives around service provision particularly with the upheaval of the restructuring of the Primary Care Trusts.

The importance of sexual health promotion in the current climate cannot be emphasised enough and it is hoped that this chapter will offer some useful tips in working with that often hard to reach group, men and boys.

AIMS

The DoH (2003b) describes the aim of sexual health promotion as 'to improve the positive sexual health of the general population and to reduce inequalities in sexual health'.

Within men's health it is important to ensure that men and boys receive the same sexual health services, information and education as women and girls. The aim of men's sexual health promotion in primary care is to access men in traditional settings, such as GUM services, and develop new, attractive and accessible community settings. These settings should aim to be 'men friendly' to encourage men to use them.

The aim of sexual health promotion is, in the main, the same for males and females. Specific aims are:

❯ to reduce rates of new and undiagnosed HIV infection
❯ to reduce rates of sexually transmitted infections
❯ to reduce unintended pregnancies
❯ to reduce psychosexual problems
❯ to facilitate more satisfying, fulfilling and pleasurable relationships.

How we deliver sexual health promotion to men and boys, however, can be different from how we deliver it to women and girls. This chapter discusses ways of working with men and boys to deliver effective sexual health promotion in primary care.

WHY SHOULD SEXUAL HEALTH PROMOTION BE AIMED AT MEN AND BOYS?

Research suggests that sexual risk-taking behaviour is increasing across the population. The Health Protection Agency (2005) states that:

> sexually transmitted infections are the greatest infectious disease problem in the UK today. Each year more than 1.5 million new episodes are seen in UK clinics for genitourinary medicine. The morbidity and associated mortality is substantial, and disproportionately affects gay men, marginalised communities and young men with high risk sexual lifestyles.

Why do men appear to be more at risk of sexually transmitted infection? Do they take more risks and if so why?

☞ **INFO**

The DoH (2003a) says 'around one in three men and one in five women aged 16–24 had multiple partners within the last year'.

Risky sexual behaviour is an activity that increases the odds of developing a sexually transmitted infection or an unintended pregnancy. These activities include underage sex, unprotected sex and having two or more sexual partners in the previous three months. Research by Meyer-Weitz *et al.* (2003) showed that men tend to seek more sexual partners over a lifetime than women, indicate a stronger desire for casual sex and report the desire for physical release and arousal as a primary motive for sex. Is this a primitive drive?

Men and boys are often linked with alcohol related risk-taking behaviour. Alcohol reduces inhibitions and physical and cognitive control, making safer sex practices less easy to negotiate. A recent survey by LM Research and Marketing Consultancy (2005) showed that a quarter of men aged 16–24 had had unplanned or unprotected sex after drinking.

It could be argued that in today's climate women and girls take just as many risks as men and boys, but we need to address the fact that sexual health services have traditionally been aimed at women and have been easier to access for women.

WHY DO MEN ACCESS THIS SERVICE?

Men and boys are becoming more aware of their sexual health and their sexual health needs. With the continuation of sexual health promotion for males many of the myths that abound around sexual health are gradually being addressed, encouraging more men to seek advice.

Relationship advice and promoting the value of respecting others also leads men to access services, as sexual health is not seen just as a woman's responsibility.

Sometimes men and boys have no choice but to access sexual health services, i.e. if symptoms are present. They may want to as they have heard that a service is being offered that is accessible, approachable, confidential and non-judgemental.

Embarrassment may be a factor; men may not feel able to go their GP.

One of the most important things is that it is FREE!

SEXUAL HEALTH PROMOTION AND YOUNG PEOPLE

The HDA (2003) states that the median age for first sexual experience is 14 for women and 13 for men. First intercourse before 16 is 30% for men and 27% for women and around 1% of 11–12 year olds are sexually active.

☞ **INFO**

Teenage birth rates in the UK are twice as high as France, three times as high as Germany and six times as high as the Netherlands. (Teenage Pregnancy Unit 1999)

Young people have the same rights to sexual health information as older people. These rights extend to young people with learning difficulties, young people living with disabilities and minority ethnic groups of young people.

The IAG (2005) believes that the more targeted and personal the sexual health information is at an early age, the more effective it is. Therefore, good sex and relationship education is vital.

Research has suggested that young boys/people are most anxious about confidentiality. The fear of parents or teachers finding out continues to deter young people from using services. Healthcare professionals owe young people under 16 the same duty of care and confidentiality as older patients, unless the professional believes that there is a risk to the health, safety or welfare of a young person so serious as to outweigh the young person's right to privacy, in which case child protection protocols should be followed. It is essential for professionals to be aware of the levels of confidentiality that they can provide.

When discussing sexual health promotion with boys there are certain other areas that should always be mentioned or certainly thought about.

A difficult area to discuss with a young boy is whether the sex they are having is consensual. It is not just young girls who are coerced into having sex. It might be that a relationship of trust may have to be built up before a young boy makes any kind of disclosure. There are far fewer cases of male abuse documented than female. It is essential to have access to appropriate agencies who specialise in male abuse. A further difficult issue is rape. Be aware both that the number of boys raped is probably higher than we think and also that you may come into contact with perpetrators of rape. There is a taboo that still exists in talking about male rape and some of these barriers may be removed if it is discussed as openly and honestly as possible. Sexual health promotion may be one arena in which it can be addressed.

Same sex feelings need to be considered. Sexual identity can be a very confusing issue for young men to deal with. Let the boys know that it is OK to talk about these feelings. Have positive images of gay men on display, try to use the term 'partner' rather than 'girlfriend', be aware that young boys may be feeling very confused, don't be afraid to discuss anal/oral sex and safety measures and ensure that local groups for young men are advertised.

BOX 5.1 Case study

We were asked to offer some sexual health promotion to a local group called BLAGY (Bradford Lesbian and Gay Youth). The group exists for 16–25 year olds. A HoM nurse initially attended one evening on consecutive weeks delivering informal presentations on hepatitis B and HIV and other sexually transmitted infections. At the end of each session the participants were given the opportunity to receive hepatitis B vaccinations. We then began to attend monthly to complete hepatitis courses. As new and different members attended each month, so the need to continue the sessions went on. We gave information about where hepatitis B vaccination courses could be completed; interestingly, one young person was sent away by his GP as he said that the young person was not at risk, contrary to guidelines.

The sessions have now become a regular part of the HoM work and offer an opportunity to engage with hard to reach individuals. The service is appreciated by the individuals as a service specific to and developed for and with them. There has been an article about the sessions in a BLAGY newsletter. It seems that a lot of the information has been put to good use and individuals say that they have developed more awareness about sexual health and keeping themselves and others safe. The individuals feel comfortable talking in this environment and will, we hope, develop confidence to access mainstream services.

Having something to offer is fundamental; in this instance, immunisations. This in turn leads on to being able to address other sexual health promotion opportunities.

This is also a good example of joint working. The sessions were arranged through relationships that were already established with a community development worker and Yorkshire MESMAC, a group working predominantly with gay and bisexual men and men who have sex with men. Finding out about local support agencies and approaching them is the best way of developing partnership working.

Sexual health promotion should not just be about providing condoms and screening. It should encompass feelings, emotions, respect and relationships. The earlier young boys are able to talk about respect and know what their emotions mean, the sooner they feel confident in dealing with and taking responsibility for their own sexual health.

With the personal, social and health education (PSHE) education in schools should also come parenting and fatherhood skills. In 2005, the number of pregnancies to under 16s was 7.8 per thousand (Teenage Pregnancy Unit 2007). Many of these pregnancies will be with boys under 16. It is essential to reiterate that fatherhood is for life and there is nothing wrong with wanting to be a good father and maintaining contact with the child if the relationship with its mother breaks down. Of course, sexual health promotion should also be working on ways of delaying fatherhood!

Schools are an obvious place where young boys have to be, so they're a good place to set up a sexual health promotion service. Liaise with school nurses, PSHE coordinators, school governors, the boys and head teachers to find out what is most appropriate.

☞ **INFO**

England has a conception rate of 41.5 per 1,000 (under 18) and 7.9 per 1,000 (under 16) (Teenage Pregnancy Unit 2006)

BOX 5.2 Case study

We were conducting sex and relationship education with each year group in an upper school. It was decided with the PSHE coordinator and the school nurse to try and set up a lunchtime drop-in session for the students in response to questions raised in the sex and relationship education (SRE) sessions. Our remit was to try and engage the boys through the drop-in, offer sexual health promotion and advice as to where the students could access free condoms, and to establish any health concerns that they might have.

The resources used in the SRE sessions were available to access in the drop-in, such as condom demonstrators, a contraceptive display kit, STI pictures etc. At the SRE sessions the students were informed of the new drop-in and it was advertised throughout the school. The drop-in was conducted in a small room next to the library. The students were allowed into the library at lunchtime and this provided a good opportunity to engage if no one was in the drop-in, allowing some time to establish rapport.

The drop-in was very successful, with the students tending to show maturity and responsibility. It was an opportunity to encourage the boys to grow in confidence and many of the boys turned up to see the HoM worker at the Lads' Room in the town centre, many asking for condoms and some taking advantage of the sexual health screening on offer.

When providing services for young people it is again important to deliver a free, confidential, non-judgemental service and to reiterate that sex is a fun, loving experience that should be enjoyed and be carried out safely.

SEXUAL HEALTH PROMOTION WITH VULNERABLE GROUPS

The issue of where and how to target vulnerable groups is not as difficult as it sounds. Outreach work involves making contact with people on their own territory and this very often applies to vulnerable groups, who may not feel able to access mainstream services but are often those most in need. Research suggests that sexual risk-taking behaviour is increasing across the population, therefore people at high risk of acquiring STIs need specific targeting, being careful not to stigmatise but recognising their particular needs.

The underlying theme for where and when to run sessions for men and boys to address sexual health promotion is to go where the men and boys meet. Be prepared to offer outreach, out of hours work, work on a client led agenda, ensuring what you are delivering is what is wanted and needed, and respect what the individuals do. Persevere, very often it takes time to gain trust and sessions may be slow to take off but word of mouth and adopting a non-judgemental, respectful attitude will pay dividends.

BOX 5.3 Case study

Outreach work has been established in male saunas in the area. These establishments cater for gay men and men who have sex with men. It is important to bear in mind that these men may be married and there may be an element of secrecy involved, therefore approach is very important.

First contact with the sauna was to provide condoms and to ensure that confidentiality was paramount. The initial visit with the owners was to raise awareness and discuss possibilities to expand services and to promote the health of the sauna users. Posters and leaflets were left for the men to read explaining that a free, confidential service was going to be offered by a male nurse on a monthly basis.

There is now a good uptake of services provided which includes condoms, lubricants, hepatitis B vaccinations, BP, blood glucose and cholesterol checks, sexual health information and advice, details of local sexual health services and a strong emphasis on safer sex practices. The *National Strategy for Sexual Health and HIV* (2001) cites gay and bisexual men as a hard to reach group at particular risk of HIV/STI, and offering outreach sexual health promotion is a way to target this group of men.

The sauna work has now become well established and pilot sessions are now being run in female saunas targeting the male customers of the women.

HOW SHOULD I MARKET THE WORK?

Men and boys need positive and proactive targeting for sexual health promotion. Specific sexual health activity needs to be developed with them if at all possible. Consideration needs to be given to ways of making sexual health services more inviting to men and boys, rather than simply trying to engage them with what is already on offer.

Positive images and messages need to be included in any literature, taking care to avoid images that may reinforce misogyny. Practical messages need to be put across, such as dispelling myths about sexual health screening for men, e.g. 'they use an umbrella device to scrape out bacteria from your willy' (it is extraordinary how many men still believe this) (Bradbeer *et al.* 2006).

Once there has been recognition about what men want and need there are several other ways in which to market sexual health promotion. It could be advertised as a confidential, free and accessible service run by men for men. It would be beneficial if it was held where men and boys are without taking them out of their way. It should be offered in an informal environment if at all possible, rather than places such as health centres where men traditionally don't go.

Bear in mind the power of the Internet, as it's principally used by men and boys.

BOX 5.4 Case study

The local information shop provides support with benefits, housing, job applications etc. for young people aged up to 25 years. It also runs a 'Lads' Room' session twice weekly aimed at young men. This is marketed as a service 'for males by males'. The male workers offer free condoms (including demonstrations), sexual health advice, information on relationships and sexual identity and referral to the STI testing service which runs alongside the Lads' Room. This is provided by a practitioner from the local GUM department. The Lads' Room facilitator explains the testing procedure (non-invasive urine testing) and discusses STIs prior to referral.

The information shop is in the centre of town, making it very easy for young men to get to, with the Lads' Room discreetly positioned at the back of the shop in an effort to maintain confidentiality. The Lads' Room has grown in success and averages 15 contacts per 2 ½ hour session.

The Lads' Room is an excellent example of how to provide sexual health promotion in a non-health setting, by taking the service to where young men meet. By using these marketing techniques it's possible to enhance the sexual health of men, young men and boys in a variety of settings.

WHERE AND WHEN SHOULD SEXUAL HEALTH PROMOTION FOR MEN BE PROMOTED?

By providing sexual health promotion in non-traditional settings, it is hoped that primary care workers will be able to help improve the sexual health of men and boys. Men and boys have traditionally been seen as a hard to reach group for many reasons. Sexual health is often seen as a woman's responsibility, or men say that they haven't got time to see a practitioner – men can always think of excuses. The *National Strategy for Sexual Health and HIV* (2001) states that:

> some groups need targeted sexual health information because they are at higher risk, particularly vulnerable or have particular access requirements. Strategies need to be developed to respond to the specific information and prevention needs of local populations.

By specifically targeting sexual health promotion at men and boys, half the population is being reached.

As with all services, it needs to be:
) wherever men and boys are
) outside normal working hours
) offered as men-only provision
) no appointment, drop-in service.

There are many places in which it is possible to offer sexual health promotion in the community:
) schools, working with the PSHE coordinator and school nurses
) youth centres and community centres
) hard to reach clients through youth offending teams, pupil referral units, local drug services, barbers' shops, male saunas
) workplaces
) pubs.

BOX 5.5 Case study

An ideal venue for sexual health promotion in the community is the local drugs agency. The agency offers a needle exchange scheme and one-to-one counselling with drug misusers. Despite beliefs, drug misusers are concerned about their sexual health and a drop-in service was set up to provide information on sexual health, contraception, hepatitis B immunisations, free condoms, leaflets etc. The drugs service advertised the fact that a male nurse would be available at certain times for a free and confidential service.

The service was slow to start but perseverance and word of mouth has resulted in a busy, popular session, which has also led to regular planned information sessions for staff and service users. Within the drug service, sexual health promotion is targeted at different populations of drug users. The main audience is heroin users but there is a steady increase of steroid users, who do not tend to see themselves as drug misusers. With the nature of the effects of steroids on the male body, gynaecomastia, impotence, shrinkage of genitals, it is an ideal opportunity to address sexual health and discuss how steroid use can affect sexual performance – the very opposite effect to the one steroid users are hoping to achieve, namely attraction of the opposite sex!

With the rapid increase of steroid users accessing the drugs project we are now developing a new project working with the Bridge project, the needle exchange coordinator and an ex-British 'natural' body building champion to deliver informed steroid information and harm minimisation to users of fitness clubs in the Bradford area.

The success lies in the fact that the service was taken to where the service users were going anyway, was confidential and was delivered in a non-judgemental, relaxed way with no pressure on the men to engage.

This also shows an excellent example of partnership working.

Sexual health promoters need to consider what needs to change to encourage men and boys to attend voluntarily and gain a positive experience. This requires a degree of imagination and creativity, taking into account what appeals to men, where to reach them and building up credibility with them.

WHAT EQUIPMENT DO I NEED?

When working with men and boys, anything that is 'free' is guaranteed to generate interest. In sexual health promotion, condoms would seem to be the obvious choice to be given free. Negotiate with condom reps and local condom distribution schemes to get as many varieties as possible. Bear in mind the need to cater for all target groups – coloured and flavoured condoms are essential when working with lads. Many condom reps will also supply other 'freebies' such as pens, mugs etc.

Condom demonstrators, contraceptive display kits and models of the reproductive systems are good for engaging clients. One of the most popular resources we use is an ejaculating condom demonstrator. The 'ejaculate' is a liquid that glows under an ultra-violet light, demonstrating the leakage of sperm prior to ejaculation. This is a useful device for demonstrating the importance of condom use in good time.

⊛ WARNING

When working with groups, it may be appropriate to show pictures of STIs. These always prove to be popular, particularly with younger males, but discretion is important – if someone has just been diagnosed with an STI, the last thing they want to see is an explicit picture showing the symptoms!

All resources need to be relevant and applicable. Leaflets are a good resource but are mainly used to reinforce messages, as opposed to actively promoting sexual health. The literature needs to be age-appropriate and written in plain and simple language. For younger boys and boys with learning needs, material with pictures may be more appropriate. All literature needs to be sensitive, as some of the issues that may be dealt with in sexual health promotion need to be addressed discreetly. Small, credit card size leaflets may be useful in this instance. Carry leaflets with you and make sure they have numbers of local services on them.

In schools, youth groups or when working with young boys, there are many good games on the market promoting sexual health. These are an excellent engaging tool and promote sexual health in a fun and easy to understand way at the same time as relaying important information. They're great for instigating conversation and breaking the ice when dealing with a potentially embarrassing subject.

There is a wealth of resources available but they need to be used by a confident, knowledgeable practitioner.

⊛ **WARNING**

Dressing appropriately is important. If you are working with a group of teenagers or trying to promote sexual health in a drugs agency, wearing a suit and tie may create a barrier and you may be seen as less approachable.

WHAT TRAINING AND EXPERIENCE IS REQUIRED?

Sexual health promotion should be delivered in a non-judgemental, respectful and sensitive manner. It needs to be provided by staff who are skilled, trained and confident to deliver this work.

Workers should have excellent communication skills, confidence and maintain clear professional boundaries. Sexual health promotion often involves dealing with very sensitive issues, such as disclosure of abuse, giving test results, discussing ED etc., so staff need to be able to support men and boys in these situations. Counselling skills are useful and child protection training is essential.

Language, especially around sexual health, can vary a great deal. It is important to maintain professionalism but at the same time people need to know what you are talking about and vice versa. Using slang words has a place but not if you are trying to gain street cred. Honesty is important here and can create a good opportunity for discussion, i.e. a conversation around different words for the same thing. Often words can be misheard – many a time in year 6 (ages 10–11) puberty talks it has had to be pointed out that a 'penis' isn't called a 'peanut'!

It can be embarrassing addressing sexual health with people, therefore staff need to be aware of their own values and beliefs and be able to access the correct training and support needed to deliver sexual health promotion effectively in groups or on a one-to-one basis.

The *Choosing Health* White Paper (2004) says that sexual health promotion will be delivered in a range of settings through a flexible multidisciplinary workforce including:

❯ Multidisciplinary teams headed by nurses.
❯ Extension of the roles of nurses, youth workers, community workers and pharmacists to include sexual health.
❯ Peer educators/youth workers.
❯ Mainstream primary care health programmes delivered by school nurses, men's health teams, health trainers, health visitors, midwives and practice nurses.
❯ More 'primary care practitioners with a special interest' working alongside sexual health experts in contraceptive, HIV and sexual health treatment services.

Staff need to have accurate, up-to-date information and relevant training in sexual health and health promotion. Knowledge of services available in the local area is essential to be able to refer or to offer alternatives to people. This knowledge is vital to enable partnership working.

Sexual health promotion in primary care is not rocket science and with the right training, the right approach and the appropriate support, can be delivered effectively by a multidisciplinary team.

SUMMARY

Aims	To reduce rates of new and undiagnosed HIV infection.
	To reduce rates of sexually transmitted infections.
	To reduce unintended pregnancies.
	To reduce psychosexual problems.
	To facilitate more satisfying, fulfilling and pleasurable relationships.
Why should sexual health promotion be aimed at men and boys?	The Health Protection Agency (2005) states that 'sexually transmitted infections are the greatest infectious disease problem in the UK today'.
	The morbidity and associated mortality is substantial, and disproportionately affects gay men, marginalised communities and young men with high-risk sexual lifestyles.
	It could be argued that in today's climate women and girls take just as many risks as men and boys, but we need to address the fact that sexual health services have traditionally been aimed at women and have been easier to access for women.
Why do men access this service?	Men and boys are becoming more aware of their sexual health and their sexual health needs.
	If symptoms are present there may be little choice but to access sexual health services.
	Embarrassment may be a factor; men may not feel able to go to their GP.
Sexual health promotion and young people	The HDA (2003) states that the median age for first sexual experience is 14 for women and 13 for men. First intercourse before 16 is 30% for men and 27% for women and around 1% of 11–12 year olds are sexually active.
	Young boys/people are most anxious about confidentiality. The fear of parents or teachers finding out continues to deter young people from using services.
	A difficult area to discuss with a young boy is whether the sex they are having is consensual. It is not just young girls who are coerced into having sex.
	Same sex feelings need to be considered. Sexual identity can be a very confusing issue for young men to deal with. Let the boys know that it is OK to talk about these feelings.
	Sexual health promotion should not just be about providing condoms and screening. It should encompass feelings, emotions, respect and relationships.

Sexual health promotion with vulnerable groups	Sexual risk-taking behaviour is increasing across the population, therefore people at high risk of acquiring sexually transmitted infections need specific targeting, being careful not to stigmatise but recognising their particular needs.
	Be prepared to offer outreach, out of hours work, work on a client led agenda, ensuring what you are delivering is what is wanted and needed and respect what the individuals do.
	Persevere, very often it takes time to gain trust and sessions may be slow to take off, but word of mouth and adopting a non-judgemental, respectful attitude will pay dividends.
How should I market the work?	Consideration needs to be given to ways of making sexual health services more inviting to men and boys, rather than simply trying to engage them with what is already on offer.
	Positive images and practical messages need to be included in any literature.
	It should be offered in an informal and convenient environment, stressing confidentiality.
Where and when should sexual health promotion for men be promoted?	Sexual health is often seen as a woman's responsibility or men say that they haven't got time to see a practitioner – men can always think of excuses.
	Services should be:
	Wherever men and boys are.
	Outside normal working hours.
	Offered as men-only provision.
	No appointment, drop-in service.
	Consider what needs to change to encourage men and boys to attend voluntarily and gain a positive experience, taking into account what appeals to men, where to reach them and the need to build up credibility with them.
What equipment do I need?	Condom demonstrators, contraceptive display kits and models of the reproductive systems are good for engaging interest.
	Have a good variety of condoms to give away. Many condom reps will also supply other 'freebies' such as pens, mugs etc.
	Leaflets are a good resource but are mainly used to reinforce messages. They need to be age appropriate and written in plain and simple language.
What training and experience is required?	Sexual health promotion needs to be provided by staff who are skilled, trained and confident to deliver this work.
	Workers should have excellent communication skills, confidence and maintain clear professional boundaries.
	Counselling skills are useful and child protection training is essential.
	It can be embarrassing addressing sexual health with people, therefore staff need to be aware of their own values and beliefs and be able to access the correct training and support.

CHAPTER 6

Weight management in the workplace

ANDREW HARRISON

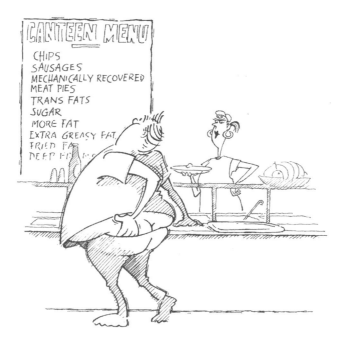

INTRODUCTION

In 2006 *Men's Fitness* magazine declared Bradford to be the fattest city in the United Kingdom. Alarmist perhaps, but it highlighted obesity as a serious public health problem and one which looks likely to escalate. Obesity is of course not unique to Bradford or the UK, it affects millions of people worldwide.

Traditionally obesity is defined by using the well established BMI indicator. The calculation of height in metres^2 divided by weight in kilograms gives a figure known as the BMI. A more practical alternative is available, in the form of BMI ready reckoners, which are both widely available and easy to use. A BMI of between 20–25 is termed healthy; 25–30 is overweight, 30 plus as obese. In practice, accurate weighing scales and height measurers are required for the test.

If it's practicality you're after, then look no further than the humble tape measure, an excellent tool which can be used to identify excess weight in men. Colour coded tape measures are available form the British Dietetic Association (www.bdaweightwise.com). Basically, if the waist measurement is 37 inches or above there is an increased health risk, while 40 inches and above indicates a high health risk.

☞ INFO

It's predicted that, if present trends continue, more than three-quarters of men in the UK will be overweight or obese by 2010 (National Audit Office 2001; DoH 2006).

WHY SHOULD MEN BE PARTICULARLY CONCERNED?

In England, more men than women are overweight or obese, 65% have a BMI of more than 25 compared with 55% of women (DoH 2003c). Male obesity is increasing much more rapidly than female obesity (British Heart Foundation, in written evidence to the Health Select Committee 2003).

Excess fat is more damaging to health when it is carried around the abdomen (Royal College of Physicians 2004). Men tend to put fat on around the stomach and upper abdomen, whereas women tend to gain weight around the hips and bottom.

This abdominal fat or central obesity is associated with an interlinked group of symptoms (type 2 diabetes, high BP, high triglyceride levels, low levels of high density lipoproteins or 'good cholesterol') that together form 'metabolic syndrome', one of the most damaging consequences of obesity.

Obesity increases the risk of developing heart disease, circulatory problems and type 2 diabetes. Obesity is also linked with significantly greater risk of several cancers, namely colorectal cancer, oesophageal cancer and kidney cancer (Key *et al.* 2004) and it remains second only to smoking as the most preventable risk factor for cancer.

☞ **INFO**

Excess weight affects men of all ages and social classes, although men in social class 1 are the least likely to be obese (DoH 2003c).

It is estimated that 14,000 male deaths each year occur in England as a direct result of obesity (National Audit Office 2001) and this may represent only a fraction of the premature deaths to which excess weight and its consequences are a contributing factor.

Obesity is top of the political agenda. The *Choosing Health* White Paper (2004), attempts to encourage people to eat more healthily, eat less and exercise more. This healthier lifestyle approach was adopted in the HoM weight management programme which aims to support men for whom excess weight is a problem, offering them advice and support to encourage healthier lifestyles. In 2005 the project received a Queen's Nursing Institute Innovation and Creative Practice Award for its work in this area of men's health.

THE HOM PROJECT

The HoM weight management project originated in community development work. Drivers at a local community centre requested help in their struggle to lose weight and a 10-week course was designed and delivered. The group continued to meet for 12 months, until numbers dwindled and the group was disbanded. However, the knowledge and skills learnt by those running the group were to prove extremely useful in the future delivery of workplace programmes.

Health-style MOTs were often used as a recruiting tool. These one-to-one consultations last 30–45 minutes and are designed to provide basic health checks and to give men the opportunity to discuss health issues in a confidential manner. Hence, overweight or obese men were offered the opportunity to take part in a workplace self-help group.

Aims:

❯ to establish weight management groups in workplace and community locations
❯ to provide these groups with ongoing support and advice to help men achieve a healthy weight
❯ to empower key members of the group to run their own weight management group independently when the initial six week course is completed.

WHERE SHOULD I RUN THE GROUPS?

Anywhere there is an opportunity.

A health promotion specialist with Bradford Council performed a vital role in initial negotiations and ensured that HoM had an opportunity to work in various Bradford Council departments.

Groups have subsequently been established in numerous workplaces and community settings, and additional groups are planned for the future.

Companies range in size from small to large-scale multinational engineering and chemical firms.

Below are some examples of existing groups and how they have evolved.

❭ Shop fitters (established 2005). The numbers have grown from 8 to 11 men. They have been successful in maintaining lifestyle changes and weight loss (*see* Appendix 6.1) and have received excellent local press coverage.

❭ Ten gardeners (employees of Bradford Council) incorporated a weekly walk into their programme and their sessions lasted for ninety minutes to accommodate this. Ten men walking through a local wood each week did receive the odd look, but it provided a further opportunity for some of the men to discuss their health concerns in a safe and relaxed environment. The group leader developed an interest in providing BP checks for members of the group and colleagues throughout his department. Any man with hypertension is referred on to his health centre.

❭ Our only mixed group (three women and nine men) exists within a large chemical firm. One particular meeting was attended by over 50 men from the company, when the group leader arranged for Professor Alan White (Leeds Metropolitan University) to deliver a formal lecture and participate in a question and answer session.

❭ A community group have recruited new members by being interviewed on radio and in the local press, and they now have 17 members. They have moved to a larger venue to accommodate the growing numbers and to provide adequate space for exercise classes.

A unique approach to health has evolved. This includes a weekly weighing for the men where each is offered support and encouragement. BP, blood glucose and cholesterol can be checked. Guest speakers are invited to present on a range of topics, including first aid, prostate awareness, heart disease and mental health. A treasurer has been elected and a nominal weekly fee of 50p is charged. One of the members is now a volunteer with the HoM project.

☆ HANDY HINT

Try to be flexible and prepared for hiccups. It can be time consuming and challenging following up MOTs in an effort to establish weight loss groups, but try to remain positive.

In reality, the planning and delivery of health MOTs did not always lead to weight loss groups being created despite sufficient numbers of men showing an interest and good opportunities were lost. Often events happen which are outside of your control and things do go wrong. For instance:

 ❯ Some businesses were keen to participate in the health MOTs, but were less willing or able to then release men on a weekly basis to attend a weight loss group. The firms expressed concern that production would be affected.
 ❯ Absence of the workplace coordinator, for example on sick leave. These people were responsible for coordinating the project, 'getting bums on seats'. When they were missing, difficulties were more likely to occur.
 ❯ Poor communication within firms, for example, nobody turned up for a course that had been planned months in advance. On another occasion, a new group had eight women and only two men, a logistical problem for a men's health initiative.
 ❯ Redundancies and a changing financial climate for businesses.
 ❯ There have been groups in the community and workplace who having completed the six week course have not wanted to continue independently.
 ❯ Community groups lack the obvious carrot of being held in work time and as a result can be more difficult to establish and maintain.

WHEN SHOULD I RUN THE SESSIONS?

The answer is simple – be flexible and run the sessions whenever you get the opportunity.

This programme is comprised of six weekly one-hour meetings. Within the workplace it is ideal if the men can attend within work time. In practice, the majority of employers have supported this, or opted for a 50:50 split (thirty minutes work time/thirty minutes employee time). On the occasions where employers have opposed this, insisting that men attend in their own time, attendance was still relatively good, with numbers ranging from four to ten.

The community courses have taken place during afternoons and early evenings.

HOW SHOULD I MARKET THE WORK?
Workplace

Health MOTs are an excellent recruiting tool for weight management groups. If it is your intention to use MOTs in this way, make it *very clear* to employers at the beginning of any negotiations and this will hopefully prevent confusion further down the line. You may even consider drawing up a contract.

One of the classic challenges we encountered occurred when employers were keen to have the MOT service and gave the impression that they would support any subsequent weight loss groups, but when the time came did not.

The method of promoting weight loss groups to men can vary. During an MOT session, names of men can be recorded (with their consent) and these details then forwarded to the workplace coordinator. The coordinators ensure the men receive any pre-course information and sort out the logistics from the company's point of view. Word of mouth, email, posters and newsletters have all been used to good effect to aid recruitment.

On other occasions, the groups may be open to all, regardless of MOT attendance.

Community

Various media sources can be used to recruit, including local press and radio.

Posters can be distributed at local health centres, libraries, community centres and swimming pools advertising the course details.

Raising the profile nationally

Articles in national newspapers, nursing journals and conference presentations, such as the HoM conference in Bradford (May 2005) and the Men's Health Forum *Hazardous Waist* conference (June 2005) have helped to get the message out, and have led to this approach being adopted and replicated in other parts of the country.

WHY DO MEN ACCESS THIS SERVICE?

❭ They do want to lose weight.
❭ It works. For some men this can be the catalyst they need to commence a healthier lifestyle.
❭ It is in work time (a huge plus factor) and does not impact on their family time or commitments.
❭ It is free, in contrast to many of the commercial slimming organisations.
❭ It is a sociable, informal event.
❭ Because of 'ear bashing' from wives, girlfriends, partners and family.

WHAT TRAINING/EXPERIENCE/SKILLS ARE REQUIRED?

A background in nursing and community development work can help. However, if you are interested, and have the time and motivation, then you can put together a similar package.

❭ A sense of humour helps.
❭ Be creative and innovative.
❭ Enlist the support of others, in particular dieticians. If you're very lucky, get a psychologist/psychiatrist on board.
❭ Record successes and failures, and modify programmes accordingly.
❭ Shadow workers already involved in the field.

Your role as the health worker is to set up groups and get them established; remember that ultimately the idea is to create groups which will be independent and require little or no input from health workers.

WHAT EQUIPMENT DO I NEED?

❭ Have copies of a weight management programme to hand when delivering MOT sessions, to show, discuss and encourage attendance in the future.
❭ Invest in quality weight scales sufficient to weigh the heaviest of men. We worked with one man who suffered the embarrassing experience of being weighed on two sets of scales at his local health centre, one foot on each set.

(The process of getting weighed can become ritualistic for many men, as it probably is for women. Anything that can be removed is removed, keys, shoes, not to mention a toilet break. The atmosphere is rife for competition, banter and humour.)

❭ A tape measure for waists
❭ A height measure
❭ BP machine and referral guidelines
❭ Cholesterol machine and strips, finger prickers, sharps bin and cotton wool
❭ A range of stationery, weekly personal weighing cards (credit card sized to fit in the pocket/wallet) and a record of the group's progress
❭ Good quality pedometers
❭ A digital camera
❭ A range of books/DVDs. In particular Haynes *HGV Man* (Banks 2005); Costain *Diet Trials: how to succeed at dieting* (2003) and the DVD *Super Size Me* (Spurlock 2004).
❭ To illustrate the amount of weight lost each week you may want to buy replica fat, but to be honest packets of lard work really well (beware – they melt!)
❭ A variety of leaflets on healthy eating, food labels, salt/fat content etc.
❭ Tea, coffee and milk (no sugar).

Note: A fee may be needed to cover the cost of some community venues.

☆ HANDY HINT

In general, men appear to prefer their weight recorded in pounds rather than kilograms, so try to ensure that any scales you purchase offer both readings. This may be tricky though with all the new EU guidelines!

⊛ WARNING

Men appear to underestimate or be in denial when it comes to their actual waist size. Ask a man his waist measurement, add four to six inches and you won't be far off the actual figure.

HOW CAN I PUT TOGETHER A PROGRAMME FOR A GROUP?

The HoM six-week programme is outlined below. Ultimately, the programme is flexible, responding to the needs and wishes of each group. For instance, when one of the men shared his weight loss secret, changing his drinking habit from over ten cans of strong lager to two bottles of wine a night, a session on alcohol was included!

The course involves a variety of topics:

) The introductory session records baseline observations: BP, blood cholesterol and glucose levels, BMI, waist measurement and 5–10% targets of weight loss are introduced. Food diaries are discussed and some men give them a try, some don't. Ideally, it helps if two workers manage the first session as it can be very time-consuming (depending on the size of the group) checking everyone's BP/ cholesterol.

⊛ WARNING

Be specific with food diaries. One diet user had been returning a completed form back to his practice nurse and all looked in order – two Weetabix for breakfast, small salad for lunch and tuna pasta for evening meal. The problem was that the tuna pasta was prepared in a washing up bowl – portion sizes had been overlooked.

) Obesity is defined and our obesogenic society explored.
) Motivation. The benefits of achieving a healthier weight are discussed and a variety of quizzes can be utilised. Successful techniques and strategies are promoted.
) Healthy eating. Many of us may feel comfortable promoting healthy eating and the balance of good health within our work. However, all the men involved in this project appeared to really appreciate and value an opportunity to question the expert – a dietician. This role was fulfilled by a community dietician employed by Bradford Teaching Hospitals Trust.
) Men develop into 'expert patients', sharing the knowledge they have gained from the sessions with new group members. On a more practical level, groups can prepare healthy snacks and fruit smoothies.
) Exercise. Frequency, type and intensity are discussed. Health promotion specialists, and in particular the *Walking for Health* coordinator for North Bradford Primary Care Trust, provide support and advice to all our groups.

☆ HANDY HINT

Find out what 'exercise on prescription' schemes are available in your area and be aware of the referral criteria.

❭ The final meeting requests course feedback. More importantly, it allows each group the time to debate their future sustainability, to nominate a group leader and to plan further sessions and levels of support.

Other points to consider

What funds are involved?

The weight management project was funded by £6,000 as part of the Queen's Nursing Institute Innovative and Creative Practice Award. This amount was to be divided between the eight groups, hence providing £750 per group. Surplus cash has been used to develop new groups. The money provided each group with sufficient funds to purchase quality scales and reimburse guest speakers and group leaders. With one exception, all of the group leaders took on this role on a voluntary basis.

The equipment purchased varied between the groups, from traditional 'health' purchases such as BP machines and pedometers to walking boots for all group members.

Groups **can** be established at minimal cost, especially if you only use a tape measure instead of weighing scales. In addition, many employers were delighted that the HoM team provided these services free of charge and they would have contributed to equipment costs.

Develop good working relationships with colleagues, dieticians and exercise advisors.

Remember any anecdotal stories that you have picked up along the way and share them with groups. Keep a record of your session plans.

Calibrate your equipment.

WHAT HAVE BEEN THE KEY SUCCESSES?

❭ Men lose weight and waist measurements decrease.
❭ New members join established groups.
❭ Effective team work from health professionals.
❭ Excellent local and national publicity promoting the project.
❭ The project is now an integral part of the HoM model for engaging with men in the workplace and it has been incorporated into the Primary Care Trust local delivery plan.
❭ The work has been replicated and developed in other areas of the country.

SUMMARY

Aims	To establish weight management groups in workplace and community locations.
	To provide these groups with ongoing support and advice to help men achieve a healthy weight.
	To empower key members of the group to run their own weight management group independently when the initial six-week course is completed.
Where should I run the groups?	In any workplace or community setting where there's an opportunity.
	Groups have been established in companies ranging in size from small/medium to large-scale multinational firms.
	Some businesses will be keen to participate in the health MOTs, but less willing or able to then release men on a weekly basis to attend a weight loss group.
	Community groups can be harder to establish as they don't have the carrot of being held in work time.
When should I run the sessions?	Be flexible and run the sessions whenever you get the opportunity.
	Within the workplace it is ideal if the men can attend within work time.
	Community courses have taken place during afternoons and early evenings.
How should I market the work?	Workplace.
	Health MOTs are an excellent recruiting tool for weight management groups.
	During an MOT session, names of men can be recorded (with consent) and these details then forwarded onto the workplace coordinator.
	Work place coordinators can use email, posters, newsletters and word of mouth to recruit.
	Community.
	Local media.
	Posters in surgeries, swimming pools, libraries etc.
Why do men access this service?	They want to lose weight.
	It works.
	It's free and in work time.
	It's a sociable, informal event.
What training/experience/ skills are required?	A background in nursing and community development work can help but isn't essential.
	Be creative and innovative.
	A sense of humour helps.
	Shadow workers already involved in the field.

What equipment do I need?	Quality scales sufficient to weigh the heaviest of men.
	A tape measure and height measure.
	BP machine, cholesterol machine and strips, finger prickers, sharps bin and cotton wool.
	Good quality pedometers.
	A range of books/DVDs.
	A variety of leaflets.
How can I put together a programme for a group?	Ultimately, the programme is flexible, responding to the needs and wishes of each group.
	Week 1 – The introductory session records baseline observations. Food diaries are discussed.
	Week 2 – Obesity is defined and our obesogenic society explored.
	Week 3 – Motivation.
	Week 4 – Healthy eating.
	Week 5 – Exercise.
	Week 6 – The final meeting requests course feedback. More importantly, it allows each group the time to debate their future sustainability.
What have been the key successes?	Men lose weight, their waist sizes decrease and groups have increased membership.
	There has been excellent local and national publicity promoting the project.
	The work has been replicated and developed in other areas of the country.

environment: *'Most of the blokes are interested to see how we all were getting on. You wouldn't associate it with a bunch of blokes.'*

Health, wealth and humour

Mark has received praise and compliments from work mates in his successful weight loss programme. However, he points out that there is a flip side to the workplace banter, and guys who haven't lost any weight get plenty of stick. There has also been a less positive aspect to weight loss that Mark never considered: *'It has cost me a bloody fortune. I had to buy not one, but two new wardrobes, after losing so much weight. The clothes I bought when I lost one and a half stone needed to be replaced when I lost another one and a half stone.'*

He now feels happy and comfortable with his weight of 13 stone.

Present status

Mark has managed to introduce exercise back in to his lifestyle. He attends the work gym three times a week, holds the current factory record for the 2000 metre rowing challenge and plays cricket on a Saturday with a local team.

Mark: *'My fitness has gone up, in fact it's probably the highest it's been in 10 years, I am especially proud of my time on the rowing machine, but I am so out of breath at the end it feels like you're breathing through your backside.'*

He still works relatively long hours, starting at 7am and finishing at 5.30pm. However he is now home at 6pm, sleeps in his own bed each night, and has time to read the kids a story. His priorities have changed:

> *I lost a lot of money (half my wage) coming inside the factory, but this was not important for me, the family is and it far outweighs the money issue, getting home to see the kids, being at their birthday parties is what it's all about, you don't get a second chance.*

He is comfortable and happy with his current health. He intends to stick with the good habits he has developed and does not want to go back to the 15 plus stone he weighed before.

Statistics in February 2006:
Waist measurement   = 37 inches (a five inch reduction).
Weight   = 182 pounds (13 stone).
Total weight lost   = 35 pounds (2½ stone).
BMI   = 26

CHAPTER 7

Smoking cessation
PETE WESTWOOD

INTRODUCTION

Smoking is the largest preventable cause of ill health and death in the UK (DoH 1998), accounting for around 114,000 deaths per year (ASH 2006). In addition, it is estimated that one in every two smokers will die prematurely, losing an average of 16 years of life (Peto *et al.* 1994 cited in DoH 1998).

These statistics need to be set alongside the news that whereas 82% of men in the UK were smokers in 1948, this has reduced substantially to 51% in 1974 (ASH 2006) and 25% in 2005 (Goddard, 2005).

☞ INFO

For the first time, there are now fewer male than female smokers in Great Britain.

In a study by Lader and Meltzer (2001), 71% of smokers expressed an intention to quit eventually, however only 11% stated that they intended to do so within the next month. Programmes aimed at action are therefore inappropriate for the majority of smokers – interventions should be stage matched with the aim of moving people through the cycle of behaviour change (Prochaska & Velicer 1997). This chapter focusses on work with clients at the 'Action' stage, i.e. those individuals who have actively committed to a specific behaviour change. Clearly, however, there is much work to be done at the national and local level to move smokers forward to this stage.

☆ **HANDY HINT**

The average smoker makes several attempts to quit before achieving success. The message is: 'Don't give up giving up!'.

The *Choosing Health* White Paper (DoH 2004b) requires public health organisations to give priority to tackling health inequalities; this is particularly pertinent to smoking, given the strong class gradient, with prevalence being almost five times greater in the most deprived groups than in the least deprived (Jarvis & Wardle 1999). Given also the gender inequality in health and the historical prevalence of male smoking, this is prime territory for public health workers who are interested in men's health.

AIMS

The broad aim of smoking cessation work with men is to help reduce the spiralling levels of heart disease, stroke, lung disease and various cancers – and as such is part of a wide spectrum of work dedicated to this goal.

There are existing DoH measures of success and databases to which smoking cessation services contribute that require basic information regarding the client and his individual quit attempt, such as the 'four-week quit rate'.

☆ **HANDY HINT**

People can sometimes feel that this work is about imposing the will of the State as part of a culture of victim blaming. Truly effective smoking cessation work, however, can only occur with those clients who themselves wish to quit.

Some useful measures of success are:
》 four-week quit rate validated by CO monitor
》 52-week quit rate validated by CO monitor
》 'harm reduction' through reduction of intake
》 short, medium and long-term health benefits.

Clients will begin to experience the benefits of quitting even in the first week. These may include:
》 reduced breathlessness
》 increased energy levels
》 improved sense of taste and smell

> improved skin colour – losing the 'smoker's look'
> increased self-esteem
> more money in their pockets.

Typical four-week quit rates for those who set a quit date are less than 50%, reducing further at the 52-week point. For those who do return to smoking, however, there is the consolation that people tend to get better at quitting with practice: *'I'm only 19 and I can't kick a ball around with my four year old without getting breathless.'* (HoM Service User)

WHERE SHOULD I RUN SESSIONS?

In short, wherever men are. In order for men to engage in health issues they often need to be on their own territory, where they are comfortable and feel unthreatened. Men may come to a health centre or hospital, but they are much more likely to engage when healthy choices are easier choices. This may mean setting up a group or meeting them on a one-to-one basis in:
> their workplace
> a school
> a pub or working men's club
> the barber's shop
> community venues, such as churches or mosques
> any other place where men meet.

The mechanism by which this work arises will vary. It may be:
> opportunistic
> planned as a natural follow-up to health MOT sessions
> requested by the host organisation
> piggy-backed onto existing work
> the result of networking and word of mouth
> the result of 'detached' work.

'My local (pub) was the last place I expected to be able to get help to stop smoking. I also got a health check!' (HoM Service User)

WHEN SHOULD I RUN THE SESSIONS?

Again, the short answer is whenever men want them. Here are some essential pointers to bear in mind.
> Can agreement be reached to run groups or one-to-ones in work time? Certainly a lot of companies are beginning to see the benefits of paying attention to their employees' health in terms of better relationships between employers and employees, reduced sickness rates and positive publicity. At the very least, can a *Stop Smoking* group be staged as an extended lunch break?

❭ Can the problem of shift work be overcome by offering a flexible service?
❭ If working in a school, can the attendees be given passes to excuse them from lessons should the session overrun a little? Young people will not readily attend a group if it takes place *after* school.

☆ HANDY HINT

Be prepared for erratic rates of attendance when running groups for young people.

❭ If the *Stop Smoking* work is as a result of health MOT work, try to strike while the iron is hot.
❭ If working in a pub, try to arrange a time when it is relatively quiet, such as an afternoon, preferably in a separate room.

☻ WARNING

Try to keep pub landlords who are sympathetic to your work onside – don't discuss with them the negative health effects of beer consumption.

'. . . it was no good trying the doctor's to see the nurse there. All the appointments were for the daytime and were booked for ages. Also, I was never going to get time off work for this; it's not like I'm ill. So when the group started at work, it was an opportunity I couldn't miss.' (HoM Service User)

HOW SHOULD I MARKET THE WORK?

As with any health promotion work, organisation is the key to success. Sometimes, though, elaborate planning simply isn't possible, especially when the work is more opportunistic in nature.

Here are some things to consider when recruiting clients for new sessions.

❭ To save yourself a *lot* of work, use organisational structures that are already in place. If in a workplace, does the occupational health nurse have a good relationship with the men that you can take advantage of?
❭ Are the communication systems up to scratch, e.g. does it take two weeks for many of the men to access emails? Does the company rely on posters or notice boards to alert men to health issues (not good)? Is there already a drive for health within the organisation, which your work can be a part of?
❭ Is the organisation actively encouraging participation from the kind of client groups that you are hoping to attract? Is there a danger that you may get a

disproportionate number of white-collar workers? Could you encourage your company contact to target the 'at risk' and 'harder to reach' men?

》 Are the employees suspicious of the motives of the company or occupational health nurse. Can reasonable confidentiality be secured and guaranteed?

》 Should there be some sort of financial contract, e.g. attendees pay a token weekly sum, or the company pays for the smoking cessation package?

》 Could there be flexibility regarding the length of the course (nothing goes exactly to plan)?

》 Could there be an option for the group to develop into a client-led support group/drop-in?

》 If the support is informal, can you guarantee the time or venue in order to deliver an adequate and cost-effective service which is easily evaluated?

⊛ WARNING

Stating that the sessions are aimed at men won't always put off women from turning up. You may even end up with more women than men. Make sure that you have a clear policy on how you will handle this if it happens.

WHY DO MEN ACCESS THIS SERVICE?

Men access this sort of service for a multitude of reasons. These may include: it's all free (or, at the very least, cheap). Don't underestimate the importance of money to men – money saved means more money to spend on other manly leisure pursuits. Nicotine replacement products, Champix and Zyban are now available on prescription, so with no hitches an entire course of treatment lasting up to 10 weeks can cost less than £20 at current prices (if the client receives free prescriptions, there is no cost at all). For a twenty-a-day habit, this compares to an expenditure of almost £400 on cigarettes at current prices over the same period.

In a similar vein, a lot of men are highly attracted to the idea of stopping smoking in work time. It's true to say that a lot of the traditional excuses for not quitting ('The Government doesn't help!' or 'The company doesn't help!') are themselves going up in smoke.

The screws are being tightened on smokers. Increasingly, employers are introducing smoke free zones or outright bans on smoking in the workplace. It's hard being a smoker these days – especially when it makes you feel like a social outcast. *'With a smoking group at work, in work's time, with the treatment on prescription and with my workmates . . . I felt I was running out of excuses'.* (HoM Service User)

The workplace is usually one of the few remaining 'men' zones (along with the garden shed and the football on Saturday). It's safe territory. Other carefully targeted venues also benefit from this feature: 'If it's OK, then men will play!'

Young men/boys have a similar experience in school settings, although there is a danger that sessions may be swamped by girls who want to quit. Teenage girls who smoke outnumber the boys and this is reflected in the numbers coming forward for help to quit. Boys in school are much more likely to opt for one-to-one sessions than groups.

☆ HANDY HINT

If you're working in a school, it's important to choose a venue that will be acceptable to young people. Rooms set away from the main school buildings where they will be less worried about being judged or reported are ideal.

WHAT TRAINING AND EXPERIENCE IS REQUIRED?

Anyone with some basic training and experience in working with groups and one-to-one sessions will be able to do this work. Here are a few tips.

❱ Try to enlist support and training from a central smoking cessation service.
❱ It may be possible to shadow another health promotion specialist who delivers a *Stop Smoking* service or find someone with suitable experience who can act as a mentor.
❱ Are you a nurse prescriber? This undoubtedly simplifies the whole process if men wish to use nicotine replacement products (NRT). If not, then try to build up credibility with local GPs so that they are likely to cooperate with your requests for NRT prescriptions.
❱ Get to know the pharmaceutical rep that has responsibility for NRT products. They are usually a mine of information, provide samples and the odd gimmicky item for attracting the attention of cautious men.
❱ Can you use the annual national *No Smoking Day* to generate interest in setting up a group? Try falling in with other agencies and then adapting their ideas to a male clientele.

☞ INFO

About 35% of smokers each year use *No Smoking Day* to take positive action about their smoking.

❱ Experience in the field is key to success – you don't learn without doing the work on a regular basis.

WHAT EQUIPMENT DO I NEED?

Nothing that you can't get into a small rucksack (should you be feeling sufficiently health-conscious to cycle to the sessions).

▶ A CO monitor (this needn't be too expensive). Use it as a motivational tool – measure the men's CO levels prior to stopping and then at least two days after they have stopped and compare the difference. They'll be impressed by the results and will begin making them a focus of competition with each other. And of course they're going to get found out if they continue to smoke – the CO monitor never lies!

☆ HANDY HINT

A CO monitor has great 'bloke appeal'. Plenty of men are unable to resist a good gadget.

▶ Collect a bag of NRT samples that the men can try out or just handle. It's also good to have some relevant 'blokey' anecdotes up your sleeve to entertain them with.

▶ Have a collection of leaflets to hand that address issues which are close to men's hearts, like how men who smoke on average have a smaller penis than men who don't, what sort of car they could afford if they kicked a £1,500 a year smoking habit and how, if they continue to smoke, they are much more likely to experience ED, even in their 30s.

HOW CAN I PUT TOGETHER A PROGRAMME FOR A GROUP?

Whilst it's good to have a plan for a typical seven-week programme (*see* Appendix 7.1), flexibility is also important so that you can respond to the specific needs of the men.

It's good to agree a joint *Quit Date* if at all possible. This will enhance the team mentality but also it will harness the underlying competitive streak in the men. One man who dropped out of a group right at the start had the misfortune to be stationed on the route to the meeting room where the group was held and was subjected to taunts of 'Weak!' from the others who were still attending.

The first two sessions should focus on motivations to stop, history taking and talking through the pharmacological options that are available. Subsequent sessions should include weekly updates and sessions dedicated to topics such as withdrawal symptoms, tips on breaking habits, what's in a cigarette? and ways of preventing possible weight gain.

Encourage banter – it can help men to relax and distract them from the reality that they are doing something which they wouldn't ordinarily countenance.

Make sure that you come across as credible. Men especially like to feel confident that you know what you're talking about.

Use 'change talk' and motivational interviewing techniques such as 'elicit-provide-elicit' and motivation and confidence scores. Be careful though not to come over as condescending.

✩ HANDY HINT

Some men may become 'expert patients' after a while and begin to actively support each other. You may even find that sometimes you need to do little more than unlock the door and switch the light on.

WHAT ELSE SHOULD I KNOW ABOUT WORKING IN SCHOOLS?

This work often presents a different set of problems. Smoking cessation work in schools is typically very difficult. Creativity in providing information is useful for helping young males to the appropriate stage of behaviour change, whereas scare tactics and dire warnings about diseases that await them are of limited value, if not counterproductive.

☻ WARNING

Sometimes it can be tempting to descend on a school and 'zap' pupils with a talk on smoking. It's best to avoid this though – a request from the young people for a visit or group run by someone who is known and trusted, or an outsider, or both, will be far more effective.

Perhaps more relevant to this client group is the idea of linking smoking to money issues and also to issues of sex and attractiveness. Certainly these topics can be utilised in a drop-in group setting.

The DoH has now released guidelines which permit the use of NRT products with over-12s. While this is indeed liberating for health professionals who recognise that some children are addicted to nicotine at quite an early age, this doesn't diminish the need to make an accurate and cautious assessment of each individual child. Many more children have issues that are centred solely around peer pressure and habit-breaking, and therefore do not require the use of NRT.

SUMMARY

Aims	The overall aim is to help reduce levels of heart disease, stroke, lung disease and various cancers.
	There are existing DoH measures of success and databases to which smoking cessation services contribute based on information such as the four-week quit rate.
Where should I run sessions?	Workplaces
	Schools
	Pubs/working men's clubs
	Barbers' shops
	Community venues (e.g. churches or mosques)
	Any other place where men meet
When should I run the sessions?	In principle, sessions can be run whenever men want them.
	Try to organise workplace-based groups or one-to-ones in work's time or extended lunch breaks.
	Pick a quiet time of the day to run pub-based sessions.
	Young people will not readily attend a group if it takes place after school.
How should I market the work?	Use organisational structures that are already in place, e.g. through the occupational health nurse in a workplace.
	See if there is already a drive for health within the organisation which your work can be a part of.
	Find the most effective communication method in the organisation, e.g. how often do people check their email, do people actually look at the notice boards?
	Could there be flexibility regarding the length of the course (nothing goes exactly to plan)?
	Could there be an option for the group to develop into a client-led support group/drop-in?
Why do men access this service?	It's free (or, at the very least, cheap). Don't underestimate the importance of money to men.
	The screws are being tightened on smokers. Increasingly, employers are introducing smoke free zones or outright bans on smoking in the workplace.
	A lot of men are highly attracted to the idea of stopping smoking in work time.
What training and experience is required?	Anyone with basic training and experience in working with groups and one-to-one sessions will be able to do this work.
	Try to enlist support and training from a central smoking cessation service.
	It may be possible to shadow another health promotion specialist who delivers a *Stop Smoking* service.
	Are you a nurse prescriber? This simplifies the process if men wish to use nicotine replacement products (NRT).
	Get to know the pharmaceutical rep that has responsibility for NRT products.

What equipment do I need?	CO monitor – these needn't be too expensive and are very useful for their 'gadget' value.
	NRT samples that the men can try out or just handle.
	Collection of leaflets addressing issues which are close to men's hearts.
How can I put together a programme for a group?	It's good to have a plan for a typical seven-week programme but flexibility is also important.
	A joint *Quit Date* will enhance the team mentality and harness the men's competitive streak.
	The first two sessions should focus on motivations to stop, history taking and talking through available pharmacological options.
	Subsequent sessions should include weekly updates and sessions dedicated to topics such as withdrawal symptoms and tips on breaking habits.
	Encourage banter – it can help men to feel more at ease.
What else should I know about working in schools?	Smoking cessation work in schools is typically very difficult.
	Scare tactics and dire warnings about diseases are not effective.
	A better approach is to link smoking to money issues and issues of sex and attractiveness.
	Boys in school are much more likely to opt for one-to-one sessions rather than groups.
	Many children have issues that are centred solely around peer pressure and habit-breaking and therefore do not require the use of NRT.

APPENDIX 7.1 SAMPLE SESSION PROGRAMME FOR A STOP SMOKING GROUP

In each session, try to encourage banter wherever appropriate. Manly humour and topics such as work and football, when employed in moderation, can really help to achieve a relaxed and 'bloke-friendly' atmosphere.

Session 1
) Introductions
) History taking – relevant medical conditions, contact details, details of previous attempts
) What help is there? – NRT, Champix, Zyban, other aids to quitting
) Quitlines
) Discuss motivations to stop smoking
) CO readings
) Agree a joint *Quit Date* (though some might want to get off to a head start before the others)
) Ask the men to consider for next week what pharmacological help they might want – patches, gum, nasal spray, Zyban* etc.

*Men using Zyban will have to see their GP as soon as possible in order to coordinate their quit date with the rest of the group.

Session 2
) Go through the options again
) Have those using Zyban started their treatment?
) Suggest practical tips for the days leading up to the *Quit Date*
) Discuss strategies for breaking habits
) Agree which NRT treatment needs to be prescribed (either by the group leader, if appropriate, or by the client's GP)

Session 3 – QUIT DAY
) Discuss withdrawal symptoms
) CO readings
) Any early problems?
) Round the table update
) LOTS OF ENCOURAGEMENT

Sessions 4–7
Topics as requested by the group, such as: what's in a cigarette?; minimising weight gain; quiz; CO readings; discuss problems/issues.

Celebration on reaching the 'four-week quit' mark.

CHAPTER 8

Erectile dysfunction and male incontinence clinics

CHRIS BRADLEY

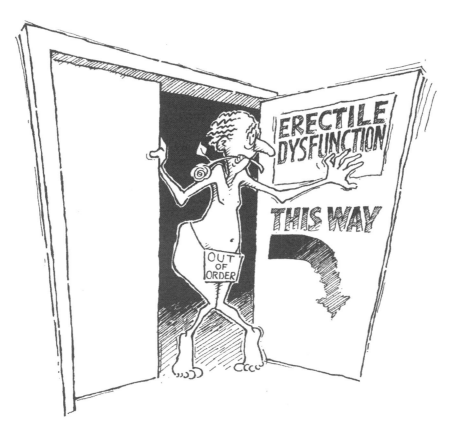

INTRODUCTION

This chapter describes the process of setting up ED and male incontinence clinics. The HoM clinics were set up and delivered by a qualified nurse with a further qualification in extended and supplementary prescribing, some specialised training in men's health and experience with a male-only caseload on secondment to a continence team. Before the HoM clinic was established there was no equivalent service available in primary care locally.

Every practitioner who reads this is likely to find themselves in circumstances and have workplace cultures, managers and individuals around them that are quite different. This will determine how best you can use this account of the HoM experience in establishing this type of service. Remember though that there is no minimum level at which to start these things, just a minimum level at which to deliver them.

AIMS

The purpose of establishing ED and male incontinence clinics based in GP surgeries/health centres is to offer a men-friendly service which will provide patients with appropriate help and advice to deal with these conditions.

Identifying potential service users and getting them through the door in the first place is also key. This requires efforts to increase referral and reporting of ED and male incontinence by getting health professionals to ask male patients the right questions.

MEN DON'T USE CLINICAL SERVICES – DO THEY?

Men are reputedly poor at reporting the symptoms of illness, especially in a proper and timely manner. Fear, delusions of indestructibility, embarrassment, ignorance, inconvenience, lack of identification with the system or setting have all been suggested as reasons why men are reluctant to access services. Sometimes men have concerns that requesting time off work to visit the doctor will be taken as a sign of weakness by bosses and colleagues. In addition, GP surgeries and clinics are often seen by men as largely feminised spaces, designed for women, children and the elderly.

☞ INFO

A study found that 71% of patients believed that ED wouldn't be recognised as a medical problem, 68% feared that discussing sexuality might embarrass the doctor and 44% of people attending urologists had ED but failed to mention it (Marwick 1999).

Men may be reluctant to report because they fear some anticipated part of the process but also because they don't know what to expect. This can be as traumatic as losing the remote control at home – they are no longer in control, and control is important to many men.

It may help to allay fears, or at least give men an opportunity to prepare themselves, if an indication of the procedures in clinic is included in the appointment mailing. A small slip of the information for the patient should always be included, so that he is as relaxed and prepared as possible, plus it helps in facilitating informed consent to the procedures. It also reduces the chances of loss of confidentiality through letters being read by others. Use phrases such as: 'A brief examination may need to be carried out that will involve loosening your clothing but does not usually require you to remove more than your outer garments. If this is not acceptable to you please inform me when you attend.'

☆ HANDY HINT

Providing patient information on a separate slip rather than in the appointment letter avoids the need to have a large number of templates or to individually compose each letter.

HOW SHOULD PATIENTS BE ASSESSED?
ED

The assessment process for this can be fairly complex, mainly for those patients who are not aware of any underlying condition that may be a likely or contributory cause, such as diabetes, hypertension, hyperlipidaemia, depression or hypogonadism. It is also commonly associated with prescription or other drugs. The first aim of assessment in these cases is to screen for these conditions, which may exist but may be undiagnosed and unnoticed by the patient. ED is also sometimes iatrogenic (caused unintentionally by a doctor), usually as a side effect of other treatments, notably surgery in the lower pelvis, most commonly prostate removal or resection. First line therapy in many of these cases is to modify the underlying condition, though this in practice rarely provides the complete answer. Assuming that coexisting conditions are under control and stable the purpose of assessment is to confirm the diagnosis from the patient's presentation.

In clinical settings it is important to have solid assessment criteria. Because we deal with people and not machines there is also scope for intuition and flexibility, though the best evidence available should always govern treatment choices. Assessment for ED is generally based upon the presenting symptoms and a comprehensive history.

The patient's experience over the previous six months is taken to be a good starting point for assessment and this can be self-assessed before clinic using a chart based on an internationally agreed scoring system. Other charts are available that give an indication of the severity of the dysfunction by rating the erection for firmness.

The most significant finding will probably be how sudden the onset of the ED was; sometimes this can be related to a particular event but in general sudden onset suggests primarily psychogenic causes whilst a gradual onset suggests a degenerative process and therefore an organic cause. If erections still occur in some circumstances this also suggests that an organic cause is less likely.

In most cases there will be a degree of both, though 80% of cases are said to have an identifiable organic cause. It is advisable to examine patients briefly, looking for abnormalities that could suggest hormone deficiency (which is rare, but not too difficult to spot if severe) or undue curvature of the penis that can affect the choice of therapy, as erections may cause damage if some form of scarring exists (this is the commonest cause of bent penises). Assessments are regularly carried out by nurses in many locations around the country because essentially they are straightforward and treatment does not depend greatly on coexisting conditions or the underlying pathology, though the need to be vigilant in looking for signs of more serious illness is constant.

☆ HANDY HINT

With modern oral medications, determining the cause may seem less important, after all medication tends to work for the majority of patients. The real point is to decide if counselling might also help, in which case a long-term solution may be possible.

Treatments and therapies, as with any condition, will not depend solely on the features of the presenting condition but also the overall state of health of the patient and any medications he may be taking. Of special note in this regard are heart conditions, which need to be stable and allow for the level of exercise required for sexual activity, which is about the same as required for gardening.

The assessment has its limitations and if further investigations are indicated then you'll need to refer back to the GP with an invitation to re-refer when these are satisfactorily completed. It may be appropriate to order certain blood tests and direct the results back to the GP.

Male incontinence

The HoM clinics started off by having a caseload of men with continence problems. Referrals soon built up and came from GPs, district nurses, nursing and care homes and hospital consultants. The main aim of assessment is to decide the type of incontinence present (very often this is strongly suggested on the referral); the main types are classified as:

❭ *urge incontinence* having to go in a hurry and sometimes not getting to the loo in time

❭ *stress incontinence* involuntarily passing urine when coughing, laughing, running etc.

❱ *mixed incontinence* a combination of the two.

These conditions are much more common in women but do occur in men. Men are far more commonly referred because they have problems with incomplete emptying of the bladder, reduced rate of urine flow and recurrent urinary tract infections. All these are commonly associated with prostatic enlargement and in the vast majority of cases this has been investigated or is under observation by a doctor or consultant. The symptoms are often included in the referral letter but need to be checked with the patient for accuracy.

⚠ WARNING

Some referrals are quite vague, especially if they come through a phone message. This is another thing to consider – is the referral procedure you plan to use suitable for the type of referrals you can expect? Naturally this could be better if there was a support worker to take referrals, assign them to individuals and ensure sufficient detail was obtained.

Patient diaries are very helpful and can be easily designed to gather the information you require. It is very helpful to know how often, how much and at what times of day or night urine is passed as this builds up a picture of bladder activity. A fairly common condition in men and women is when the bladder becomes overactive causing urge incontinence or extreme urgency that can control how far people go from their homes without a map of available toilet facilities. Fortunately, this is a treatable and curable condition not, as has been in the past, a matter of wearing incontinence pads or staying at home. There are good medicines, self-help strategies and, for those more resistant to treatment, surgical procedures that can alleviate this distressing condition. The latest procedure involves Botox injections into the bladder by a urologist to partially paralyse the muscle and reduce urgency and frequency.

WHY DO MEN ATTEND?

In the first instance men are often embarrassed to be asked about the very personal issue of ED that they may not have discussed before. After that they tend to be relieved that at last they have been able to discuss it; this seems to apply even to those who do not want any intervention because they have adjusted their lives to being comfortable with celibacy.

Many men who come to clinic have conditions that are the result of a prostate enlargement, and the nuisance symptoms are what makes them report to the doctor, the commonest being having to get up repeatedly during the night to go to the toilet. This is an ideal opportunity to start asking about other areas of health, especially those such as ED that are also seen as embarrassing and difficult to talk about. Lower urinary tract symptoms (called LUTS by urologists and urology nurses) such as those described in men can have the same causes as in women, but in men they need further investigation because of the common link to prostate disease. Because most of our referrals come from GPs and consultant urologists this has usually already been investigated to ascertain the nature of the prostate disease, but again this needs checking. All the conditions are treatable by various methods, but the aim in the men's health clinic is to alleviate or find ways to manage the symptoms in partnership with the patient.

WHAT SHOULD I KNOW BEFORE STARTING UP A NEW CLINIC?
Who will come

Decide who will access your clinic and how they will know where you are and how to get all the way to the door without having to ask. Men hate asking the way and this is likely to be compounded if they need to know the way to a clinic. Though there is an age correlation among those who experience these symptoms, neither is age-dependent nor inevitable. Between the ages of 40 and 70 your chances of having a severe problem with erections triples because the chances of you getting one of the diseases that cause these problems increases. At 40 years old about 5 men in 100 experience severe erection difficulties and because of the reluctance to report such things the figures are all estimated based on the best knowledge available, but could be greater or less. Some estimates vary widely.

It helps to decide on treatments offered if you can have at least one meeting with the man with his partner present. The partner's attitude to restarting sexual activity may be at variance with the patient's own and this should be investigated as there may be a physical reason; for example, intercourse could have become uncomfortable due to the woman's body changing, an experience of some women during the menopause. It may be that she or he was not so keen even when erections were possible and is relieved that intercourse is no longer a part of the relationship. Sometimes it may be possible to offer helpful suggestions or start couples toward discussing this if they have never done so, whilst for others it may become apparent that specialist counselling is needed to help with some of the relationship concerns raised.

⚠ WARNING

Unless you are trained in counselling, even a relatively low level exploration of relationship issues can become uncomfortable and requires tactful, sensitive handling.

Planning is of the essence

You don't need to be the world's best planner but to start a completely new clinical service requires a firm idea of what that will entail. The first idea may need to be adjusted and amended several times before the final project takes shape. Speaking to others who have done something similar is invaluable. We used contacts supplied by a pharmaceutical rep and phoned around some clinics within daily travelling distance to ask if we could visit. These visits raised many important issues, not only because the people were enthusiastic about the idea, but because they also knew some of the pitfalls or requirements which had yet to be considered.

> Clinical supervision – how available was it if there were no other nurses at any level with the same interest within the PCT?
> Protocols and guidelines – who would write these and who would check and sign them off?
> What referral pathways would be in place?
> What could be done to overcome resistance from local GPs?

The act of putting together a business plan helps to focus on what you want to do and why.

☆ HANDY HINT

If you need to improve reporting in your area, district and community nurses could be a good place to start. Make them aware of the service, how to refer, when the clinics are held and in what localities and above all the specific questions they will need to ask as part of their assessment.

The end result of a man visiting the clinic should always include an improvement in the situation from the patient's perspective. Review documentation in the patient's record should reflect if this is the case. A simple tick box that says: 'The patient feels that he is making progress' with alternative choices of 'no', 'some' or 'good' progress would be a start, and will transfer to electronic records and templates easily when the need eventually arises.

Know your subject

Most nurses would only consider starting a clinic if they had either a skilled accomplice or some relevant training, experience and skills. This is partly because of the sensible requirements of their professional code of conduct designed to ensure patient safety, but also because most are acutely aware of how difficult life can be for nurse and patient if all that is on offer is basic advice and referrals to others – in other words, no improvement in previous service provision.

☆ HANDY HINT

Being a man may help in running the clinic but it's important to remember that the model of manhood that you aspire to is not the only valid one around; Lennox Lewis, Graham Norton and *New Look* magnate Tom Singh are all successful men, though they all no doubt have their own ideas about what being a man is all about.

If you make your plans far enough in advance it is possible to examine carefully what mix of knowledge and skills you are likely to need, though a supportive continuing development working environment is then essential to gain experience without undue risk. Research it, go on courses, talk to others in the field, visit clinics, study it and understand men's lives by reading some of the literature about and by men. For working in the field of ED the only accredited training course is NEED (Nurse Education in ED), which can be accessed via the Royal College of Nursing (RCN). If you plan to provide a complete one-stop service you will also need to have a Nurse Independent/Supplementary Prescriber (V300) qualification, as well as being recognised as a commissioned service operating under local agreement. Other than this you may need to use supplementary prescribing procedures

Use all the resources available to you to find out, be informed and become as much of an expert as you can (but in general try not to act like one). No one, not even the law, expects you to be the world authority, but you will need to know enough about your subject to be safe and effective and make a strong case for being allowed to attempt to improve the service for men in your area. As a minimum you should always know these two things:
〉 as much about the condition as possible and
〉 the limits to your knowledge and therefore clinical input.
This could mean writing a clinical guideline or a set of rules to govern your level of input and getting it agreed by others. This can be difficult if there is no one else in your clinical group who has the same interest or expertise. There is, however, support available from other areas. Worth considering are local consultants – many have now embraced the idea of nurse led services taking some of the strain out of stretched specialist facilities. GPs with special interests exist in most areas for a wide range of conditions. These GPs are generally up to date and enthusiastic as the role has often developed around their particular interest. Other sources of help include those who have done this type of work before, though you may need to look outside your own location or PCT.

Identifying ED
One man's meaning when he says 'I have impotence' can be very different from what another man describes using the same words. Because it is not used in

everyday social parlance, 'impotence' has many meanings to different people. From the nurse's point of view it is best to have an idea of some of these popular descriptions and misconceptions. The British Medical Journal *Best Treatments* website (www.besttreatments.co.uk) describes the main errors men make when thinking they have ED: they may mean such things as premature ejaculation, infertility or loss of libido and these are different problems not helped by ED treatments.

☣ WARNING

Avoid making assumptions. It's often said that men won't talk about their health but they will and do, given the right conditions. There are lots of mistaken assumptions about men, some of them perpetuated by men themselves. It's a very good idea to check the meaning of what you are being told when you speak to men.

There is help available for men experiencing these other conditions; it is worthwhile knowing who and where to refer to as they will almost certainly occur eventually. Premature ejaculation is occasionally linked to a medical condition that needs treating but is far more often a matter of improving control of the situation. There are techniques that can be taught and the situation can be improved for some men by using a constricting ring, similar to those used by men who can't sustain their erection long enough for satisfactory sexual activity.

Talking about sex with adults

When defining ED the phrase 'sexual activity' rather than 'sexual intercourse' should be used, as the latter is a rather limiting expression that makes an assumption about how the individual may wish to use his erection. If you are not comfortable considering and discussing other aspects of male sexual activity than heterosexual intercourse then perhaps this is not the best area in which to develop your career or expertise. Having said that, it gets easier the more you do it and it is important that you are quite relaxed about it when assessing patients, so training and practice do help.

It has been suggested that one reason this is such an unreported condition is that doctors and nurses may be reluctant to ask the right questions, although this seems a bit odd considering the questions we do sometimes need to ask. This illustrates the special importance that we put on matters sexual. If you do not work in this field but want to know the basic questions to ask your patients/clients before referral, remember that the main thing is the need to be very specific; nurses have been heard to ask 'Do you have a satisfactory sex life?' or 'Can you have sex OK?'. 'How is your sex life?' sounds more like an intimate social enquiry than a medical one.

Usually it's best to be direct by saying something along the lines of 'We often find that men who have your medical condition have difficulty getting or keeping an erection, are you experiencing any difficulties in this respect?' This may sound a bit formal but you can alter the exact wording of what you say according to how well you know the patient and the degree of rapport that exists between you.

☆ HANDY HINT

It could simply be a question of including one question on assessment paperwork for many other conditions, especially those that indicate an increased statistical risk of ED.

How important is the location of the clinic?

Bad news for estate agents perhaps but you'll probably find that location is not such an important issue if men are seeking a place to discuss *personal* health issues, rather than an MOT health check, for example, where location can be important. When it comes to providing clinical services, the rules seem to change. Men choose where they are comfortable by association and what they want from it. For discussing health concerns the criteria seem to be confidentiality, comfort, not being asked any personal questions except in the safety of a clinical interview and confidence in the professional providing the service. That is where the issue of dress code comes in, as many men seem to have more confidence in professionals in suits, probably because that is what they have come to expect over the years.

Most people would rather not disclose their medical details to their neighbours and confidentiality is not so easy to achieve as may at first appear. GUM clinics that broadly speaking operate with similar problems in achieving total confidentiality use all manner of methods to maintain anonymity of the setting and those who attend, but many do not appear to work as well as they might. Using a clinic letter such as 'Clinic J' looks good but soon everyone knows the code in a local hospital, whether they use that service or not. It might be better if the letters were rotated in some way so that different disciplines shared all the letters. An excellent idea from GUM services which was adopted for the HoM clinics is that men can attend outside their own area if they wish, which is another advantage of having clinics in several localities.

HoM clinics were run at three different locations – two in health centres and one in a cottage hospital. Keighley and Airedale PCT covers a large area with only a few small towns and lots of villages. The three locations chosen cover the main centres of this area. Plans to expand will be handled in the same way. Patients weren't restricted to any particular venue, as if they want to be seen more quickly or away from where they might bump into neighbours they would often travel to a different place if they could. The electronic records system allowed access to all their records from any of the locations.

How can I find potential service users?

Potential service users suffering from unreported conditions are out there waiting to be asked. Incontinence following surgery is well reported within the system but the type that comes on gradually over a long period of time is probably much less so. GPs took quite a time to stop asking the HoM team to see people with treatable conditions and 'help them out with some pads'. The treatments are often not medical or surgical, but they do often work; such measures as pelvic floor muscle exercises (Kergel exercises) and bladder retraining, sometimes in combination with a short course of anticholinergic medication can do wonders. Incidentally, Kergel exercises can also help with ED, especially if it is not too severe. New non-medical prescribing rules from May 2006 have improved the range of options for patients in nurse led clinics.

☆ HANDY HINT

The assumption that men will not pay the private prescription charge is just that and many of these men do qualify for free prescriptions under the rules.

The main battle is in getting men to admit to a problem, especially when the problem affects what to many epitomises what it is to be a man – their biological identity. Of the men who were asked directly by the HoM nurse if they had a problem getting or keeping an erection, well over half affirmed that they did; many said that they had not been asked before and had had a problem for many years. The usual line to take is: 'We find that the condition you have/treatment or surgery you have had/ medication you are taking, quite often causes problems with erections. Do you have a problem getting or keeping your erections?' Of course, the questions that follow are just as important: does it trouble them? (it doesn't always), do they want help with it as several treatments are available? etc.

If you can get doctors and nurses asking the right questions then there will be more than enough men coming forward whose conditions were previously hidden.

How do I get men to attend?

Men sometimes don't attend for very practical reasons. They are in full-time work and time off is not easy to get without good reason. 'Good reason' generally involves explaining in some detail to the boss and colleagues what the problem is. This objection was countered quite early on in the HoM project, when running well man health check clinics, by sending out appointment letters that contain no reference to illness, just an invitation to attend for a health check – official, well typed, on NHS GP practice or health centre note paper, giving it all the credibility necessary without suggesting illness or weakness. The wording of letters needs a lot of consideration as they need to inform the patient without informing his boss, who may demand proof of an appointment. A sample of those used by HoM is included at the end of the chapter. The original invitation to attend for HoM health and lifestyle checks in a GP surgery seemed to hit the right note as there were few non-attenders. To test its transferability, it was duplicated for use in a different surgery where the case-load was mainly made up of men from the local Pakistani community and the result was the same – men attended.

The lesson from this is simple, men need to be invited by formal letter to attend, it saves them having to make their excuses, and as they did not ask for the appointment it cannot possibly be 'their fault'. Try to stick to the principle of not suggesting or detailing illness, even though the clinics deal only with men who have an identified health problem.

✆ WARNING

It can be hard to change some operational practices, even the wording of letters, without ruffling a few feathers: 'I've a couple of suggestions for keeping our team at the cutting edge of this type of service' might work better than 'It's time we reviewed our paperwork because I can see a few serious flaws'.

The key to attendance in the HoM health check clinics in GP practices seemed to be that:

❯ Men were invited by letter to a set appointment. They therefore did not have to explain the need for time off to their boss, friends or families.

❯ They provided plenty of time to think about and talk about their health without needing to justify their visit.

Surgeries may not have been in a place where men would choose to hang out but the conditions for confidential discussion were assured. If you ask men whether they would rather talk about a troublesome health condition in the back room of the local pub or in a specially set up local clinic they will choose the latter.

When is the best time to run clinics?

It would be great if the answer was 'when men most want the service', but of course it doesn't quite work like that – it would be impossible to accommodate them if they all wanted to come in at 7.30 in the evening. Many of the men are post surgery, or not in full-time work and the best that can be offered is a degree of choice and flexibility. Patients can be invited in the initial letter to phone and change appointments to more convenient times for them, although sometimes this may involve working at times outside your usual hours. If you have a colleague working in the same clinics you could perhaps rota some weekend or evening clinics, though obviously this isn't possible if the centres you're using have limited opening times and no receptionist after 5 p.m.

What makes a good venue for running a clinic?

A suitable venue will have:

❭ Some space that's totally private, with an examination couch and basic clinical facilities.

❭ A waiting area close by is useful if you don't have another person to go and call patients in, as open clinic rooms can't be left unattended because of the risk of unauthorised entry, loss of confidentiality and harm to others.

❭ A reception area where patients can ask for directions. In the invitation letter, patients can be instructed to ask for you by name to avoid embarrassment (if you're working in a clinic which is small enough to allow this). If the receptionist is welcoming this helps to make the patients more relaxed before they go in, but sadly, as in every occupation, there are the good and the not so good.

☆ HANDY HINT

If you're lucky enough to have a waiting room which is just for your patients you can put out a bit of 'male' reading.

Carrying out home visits will allow you to meet people in their everyday surroundings, where they are relaxed and in charge. The HoM team did this when teaching men to self-catheterise, as it wasn't much use if a man could do this successfully in clinic but his own bathroom was a cramped space with a difficult layout.

How long should sessions be?

You'll need about an hour for an assessment for either erection problems or incontinence. If a man presents with both you can make a further appointment and deal first with whichever problem he sees as more important. For follow-up the appointment time generally reduces to about half an hour, but play it by ear as some men want to talk for longer or have more complex issues to discuss. Ideally, you should try to allow an hour for appointments with the patient's partner present, but in busy clinics this may not be possible and it depends on the stage which you've reached in your discussions. It is important to give patients some indication of the time limits before they arrive.

The time taken to set up and wind down a clinic should not be underestimated. Everything needs to be as ready as possible beforehand and put away at the end. Unless you are very lucky you will also have your own letters to compose and possibly also to type. This takes more time than you may think. It helps to look for an appointment slot and send out the letter as soon as you get the referral, and to arrange repeat appointments (unless there is a need to leave things open-ended, such as when asking the patient to report progress) whilst you have the patient with you.

☆ HANDY HINT

It may be appropriate to have further training in using the electronic records system, but if the computer or its network has a reputation for disobedience you might want to back up as much as you can with a PDA (Personal Digital Assistant) and paper records.

SUMMARY

Aims	To establish ED and male incontinence clinics based in GP surgeries/health centres.
	To increase referrals and reporting of ED and male incontinence.
Men don't use clinical services – do they?	Men may be reluctant to report because they fear some anticipated part of the process but also because they do not know what to expect.
	It may help to allay fears or at least give men an opportunity to prepare themselves if an indication of the procedures in clinic is included in the appointment mailing.
How should patients be assessed?	*ED:*
	The assessment process can be fairly complex, especially where patients are unaware of any underlying condition that may be a likely or contributory cause.
	In clinical settings it is important to have solid assessment criteria.
	Assessment for ED is generally based upon the presenting symptoms and a comprehensive history.
	In general, sudden onset suggests primarily psychogenic causes whilst a gradual onset suggests a degenerative process and therefore an organic cause.
	Male incontinence:
	Men are most commonly referred because of problems with incomplete emptying of the bladder, reduced rate of urine flow and recurrent urinary tract infections. These are commonly associated with prostatic enlargement.
	Patient diaries are useful for gathering the information you require. It is very helpful to know how often, how much and at what times of day or night urine is passed as this builds up a picture of bladder activity.

Why do men attend?	Many men have conditions that are the result of a prostate enlargement and the nuisance symptoms are what makes them report to the doctor, the commonest being having to get up repeatedly during the night to go to the toilet.
	Services offered should fill a gap or improve on what is available from the patient's point of view e.g. more accessible, shorter wait and longer consultation time.
What should I know before starting up a new clinic?	Speaking to others who have run similar services is invaluable and will probably raise issues which you haven't thought of.
	If you make your plans far enough in advance it is possible to examine carefully what mix of knowledge and skills you are likely to need, though a supportive continuing development working environment is then essential to gain experience without undue risk.
	Decide who will access your clinic and how they will know where you are and how to get all the way to the door without having to ask.
	It helps to decide on treatments offered if you can have at least one meeting with the man with his partner present.
	The end result of a man visiting the clinic should always include an improvement in the situation from the patient's perspective.
Identifying ED	One man's meaning when he says 'I have impotence' can be very different from what another man describes using the same words.
	Men may describe such things as premature ejaculation, infertility or loss of libido as ED.
Talking about sex with adults	In the definition of ED the phrase 'sexual activity' should be used rather than 'sexual intercourse'.
	It's been suggested that one reason that ED is so under-reported is that doctors and nurses are reluctant to ask the right questions.
	It's important to be very specific and direct.
How important is the location of the clinic?	Location is not such an important issue if men are seeking a place to discuss personal health issues.
	The main issues are confidentiality, comfort, not being asked any personal questions except in the safety of a clinical interview, and confidence in the professional providing the service.
	It's best if patients aren't restricted to one particular venue as some will prefer the most convenient location whereas others will prefer to go to an area where they're less likely to bump into people they know.
How can I find potential service users?	Potential service users suffering form unreported conditions are out there waiting to be asked.
	The main battle is in getting men to admit to having a problem.
	If you can get doctors and nurses asking the right questions then there will be more than enough men coming forward.
How do I get men to attend?	Men sometimes don't attend for very practical reasons. They are in full-time work and time off is not easy to get without good reason.
	Men need to be invited by formal letter to attend – it saves them having to make their excuses.
	Confidentiality needs to be assured.

When is the best time to run clinics?	In an ideal world patients would have total freedom in when to use the service but of course this isn't practical in reality.
	The best that can be offered is a degree of choice and flexibility. Ultimately you'll be restricted by the opening hours of the health centre in which you're operating.
What makes a suitable venue for running a clinic?	Some space that's totally private, with an examination couch and basic clinical facilities.
	A waiting area close by.
	A reception area where patients can ask for directions, preferably with a friendly receptionist.
How long should sessions be?	You'll need about an hour for an assessment for either erection problems or incontinence.
	Ideally, you should try to allow an hour for appointments with the patient's partner present.
	Explain in the patient's letter how long you expect the assessment to take.
	The time taken to set up and wind down a clinic should not be underestimated.

APPENDIX 8.1 SAMPLE CLIENT LETTER

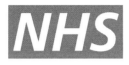

CONFIDENTIAL

Dear

You have been referred to the clinic and I am writing to let you know that an appointment has been made for you at . . . on . . . at . . . Please come to the reception area at . . . and say that you are here for an appointment with . . .

Could you please fill in the enclosed chart before you attend the clinic and bring with you a fresh sample of urine and details of any current medication. Your initial appointment will last for up to one hour.

We have an interpreting service available; please let us know as soon as possible if you would like an interpreter present for your appointment.

To enable us to provide you with the best care we will be asking your GP to allow us to see your medical records, and sharing our records with him/her. If you have any objections to this please inform me as soon as possible.

If your clinic appointment is inconvenient please contact me on . . ., to arrange a more convenient time. If the answer machine is on leave your name and telephone number clearly so that I can contact you though this may not be within the same day.

Yours sincerely

Men's Health Nurse

CHAPTER 9

Targeting ethnic minorities

MEHZAR IQBAL AND ANDREW HARRISON

INTRODUCTION

Ethnic minority groups have been found to generally have poorer health, poorer access to health services and are less satisfied with health services than the majority white population. Bringing tailored services directly to ethnic minority communities therefore has a key role to play in reducing health inequalities and inequities in access.

The population of Bradford has grown steadily over the last 100 years and it is expected that over the next five years there will be a significant rise in black and minority ethnic (BME) communities relative to a decline in the white British population. This growth of BME communities is occurring partly because the influx of new immigrants to Britain tends to favour established communities and also because BME families tend to be larger.

HoM have worked very successfully with local mosques in setting up health sessions. The first time we went to a mosque and asked to do a sexual health session they said 'What?! Oh, no, no, no, this is a mosque. This is a holy place.' Once reassurance had been given that the session was going to discuss prostate and testicular cancer rather than sexual intercourse, however, they were happy for us to come in. Sessions have also been run on general health, drugs and anti-bullying.

☞ INFO

The 2004 *Health Survey for England* (2005) found that among most ethnic minorities there does not appear to be a clear association between obesity and specific health problems such as diabetes and CHD. Men in most

> ethnic minority groups had markedly lower obesity rates than the general population.

In November 2003 we held a mosque *Stop Smoking* event in association with the smoking cessation team. This involved taking a specially decorated bus to a popular mosque (on a Friday, as this is the mosque's busiest day). The aims were to raise awareness of the link between smoking and ill health, help people to stop smoking and provide support and access to the smoking cessation services available. Leaflets in both English and Urdu were distributed and the event was attended by a large number of people, with 20 subsequently stating that they were committed to stopping smoking.

Working in partnership with the Prostate Cancer Charity and other local Bradford organisations, HoM workers took part in a charity dominoes tournament aimed at increasing awareness of prostate cancer among the African Caribbean community. African Caribbean men are three times more likely to develop the disease than other races. The tournament was fiercely contested by teams drawn from local associations and after a battle royal a Prostate Cancer Charity Cup was presented to a packed Dominica Association in Bradford. The event also included an open day in support of *Black History Month*, featuring the island of Dominica and its culture. There was wide selection of Caribbean cooking and entertainment was provided by a popular steel band.

THE HOM *BARBER SHOP PROJECT*

This chapter focusses on the nationally acclaimed HoM *Barber Shop Project*, which provides a good illustration of how to deliver a community based service targeted towards a particular ethnic group. The project was set up by an HoM nurse to target South Asian men, delivering health checks in a barber shop which also served as an informal community centre for many of the customers who met there to chat or read the newspapers.

The team offered health checks and advice to men who came into the shop and what began with a fortnightly commitment of a nurse and a bilingual health support worker expanded over time to a weekly health drop-in, with advisors from both Bradford District *Stop Smoking* service and sexual health clinic. With eight of the HoM team committed to this particular project, it became one of our largest ongoing initiatives.

AIMS

Targeted interventions such as the *Barber Shop Project* aim to tackle barriers to accessing services by taking health services directly to the target community.

The broader aim of this kind of work is to reduce health inequalities. Statistics compiled by the Commission for Racial Equality from the 1999 Health Survey for England and the 2001 Census show that:

❭ Asians and Black Caribbeans are more likely to suffer from diabetes than the general population.
❭ Pakistani and Bangladeshi men have rates of CVD about 60% to 70% higher than men in the general population, while Chinese men have lower rates.
❭ 44% of Bangladeshi men, 39% of Irish men and 35% of Black Caribbean men report being smokers compared with 27% of men in the general population. Indian (23%) Pakistani (26%) and Chinese (17%) men are less likely to report being smokers.
❭ 19% of Bangladeshi men report chewing tobacco.
❭ White Irish men are more likely than any other ethnic group to drink in excess of the recommended limit (58%). All other ethnic minority groups are less likely than the general population to drink in excess of the recommended limit.

WHERE SHOULD I RUN SESSIONS?

An appropriate location will have the following characteristics:
❭ Basically anywhere there is an opportunity.
❭ A non-healthcare setting located within the target community and open at times when potential service users will be able to attend.
❭ An informal but confidential setting will enable men to be more open-minded about engaging with health workers, as there will be no clear protocol or process to be observed by them.
❭ A male dominated/male friendly setting – men will be more open to engage with the service if they are able to observe other men doing the same. Also, they will not have to deal with issues which may potentially affect their perceptions of their own masculinity in the presence of the opposite sex.

The barber shop chosen for the HoM project was in an area that has a substantial number of residents of South Asian origin. The owner had worked in the area for over 15 years and the shop was strictly men only.

The HoM nurse realised the potential. He regularly drove past the venue, noted how busy it always appeared to be and simply made the decision to call in for a haircut and talk to the owner about the possibility of delivering men's health services. It was as simple as that.

The owner accepted. He was the first to have a health check and other men in the shop followed his lead. He genuinely wanted to help the local community and realised that the delivery of an additional free service in his shop could favour his business.

⚠ WARNING

Sometimes with this kind of work compromising on privacy and confidentiality is unavoidable. The barber shop easily became crowded but a separate room wasn't available. If a sensitive issue arose, the HoM worker would talk to the man outside on the street.

WHEN SHOULD I RUN THE SESSIONS?

Sessions need to be run at times when potential service users will be able and willing to access them – this will of course vary depending on who you are primarily hoping to attract; whilst daytime sessions will be most convenient for some, others will only be able to attend in the evenings. Basing a service in an establishment which is already well-attended by your target audience will increase the chances that the people that you want to reach will be there when you are, even if they are totally unaware of your service before they arrive.

Of course, it is of little use being in the same place at the same time as your potential service users if they are unable to hang around long enough to use the service. For the *Barber Shop Project* it was decided to run sessions at the shop's busiest time, as this would be when waiting times would be high, giving those who were waiting for a haircut sufficient idle time to make use of the service (boredom can be a great motivation for people to engage with something which might otherwise have failed to capture their attention).

The work developed gradually. What began as a monthly session developed into a fortnightly commitment and then became a regular 2–3 hour session. This was purely based on the needs of the men and the owner, who was happy for men to come into his shop to access our services *without having a haircut*.

HOW SHOULD I MARKET THE WORK?

The support of a key figure was vital. In the barber shop it was the owner, in the workplace it would be a named coordinator. He would promote our services by word of mouth to men in his community.

The project was promoted through a variety of sources, these included:
) libraries
) community centres
) convenience stores
) mosques
) takeaways and restaurants
) taxis
) pubs and cafes
) local radio
) local and national press
) nursing journals
) filming by the HDA of the barber shop in action.

Once suitable sites have been identified, a project can be marketed quite simply by having a presence there and 'being seen to be doing'. Flyers or posters may also help with basic information describing what is on offer, times, dates and contact numbers.

If you're setting up a service in a venue where potential users will not already be, marketing becomes even more important. In some cases it might be appropriate to try to entice people with the prospect of free food, drink and transport.

WHY DO MEN ACCESS THIS SERVICE?

Men accessed the barber shop service because it was:

❭ free
❭ marketed in their comfort zone (the community setting)
❭ delivered on their terms
❭ delivered in their comfort zone
❭ delivered by someone with credibility in the community.

This kind of service offers an alternative source of health advice for men who may:

❭ not be registered at a GP surgery
❭ fear rejection from a GP
❭ feel embarrassment about taking what they perceive to be a trivial problem to the GP
❭ have potential health problems but poorly defined symptoms with which they feel unwilling to visit the GP
❭ lack understanding of the UK health system.

When setting up services targeted at ethnic minorities, it's useful to bear in mind some of the key issues which have been found to affect how often different ethnic groups access health services. These include:

❭ lack of understanding of health services
❭ language and literacy difficulties
❭ cultural differences (problems were encountered and overcome regarding the distribution of condoms)
❭ different needs of different populations
❭ location of service delivery.

Advice which emerges from a friendly environment and a person with community credibility has a greater chance of being acted on, even if it involves further trips to the much avoided primary care centre or GP practice.

> *Initially I did not know what to make of them. But when I saw other men talking to you and having a health check I thought I may as well get myself checked out. I work six days a week in a restaurant and I do not have time to see the doctor. I speak Urdu and he speaks English. My wife works; I know my GP tries his best but I do not feel comfortable going on my own.* (HoM Service User)

WHAT SHOULD BE INCLUDED IN A TYPICAL SESSION?

This will of course depend on the specific nature of the service that you wish to provide and the needs of the men. Devising a standard format will enable you to make the most efficient use of what may only be a short time with each individual and will also help the men to know what they can and can't expect to receive. Whenever possible, try to utilise health resources which will be best suited to the environment.

The barber shop health checks were structured as follows:

) general introduction
) basic health checks, which included BP, pulse, waist measurements, BMI, blood sugar and cholesterol (CO levels could be checked if necessary)
) general conversation about lifestyle and healthy eating
) advice and/or referral
) if appropriate, information leaflets were distributed.

☆ HANDY HINT

BMI can be a useful tool to open up discussion on diabetes. It also serves partly to meet men's expectation of being physically examined.

When a man would come in for a haircut or just for a social meeting either:

) the barber would ask if the man wanted to see the HoM worker
) the man would ask what was going on and then ask if he could have something done
) the HoM worker would gently ask him if he wanted to, say, have his BP taken
) the man was on a repeat visit, e.g. to have his blood sugar checked.

The approach was such that the man could decline without embarrassment e.g. the barber might make the approach in Urdu so that the man could decline without the HoM worker being directly involved.

At the end of the examination if there were any problems, such as a raised BP or blood sugar level, the man was given a referral note for his GP. *'This is the best hair cut I have had – apart from looking good I now know why I am going to the toilet a lot. I thought I was thirsty because of the curries I was eating and drinking coke.'* (HoM service user)

HOW EASY IS IT TO REPLICATE THIS TYPE OF PROJECT?

An important issue is whether the model used with the *Barber Shop Project* can be replicated elsewhere. There are several important factors here:

❯ The barber was a part of the community in a way that many barbers no longer are. It is a traditional barber's shop that is now probably specific to certain communities with a regular clientele.

❯ It was a place to meet sociably, not just for the purpose of having a haircut; this was a result both of cultural factors and the personality of the barber.

❯ The arrangement to use the shop was the result of a personal relationship and the initiative of the HoM worker who made it. There was a high degree of cooperation between HoM workers and the owner of the shop.

⚠ WARNING

We attempted to set up similar projects in white barber shops, but with little success. Often the owners feared that a 'full' shop would deter people from coming in off the street as this would mean longer waiting times. They perceived (with good reason) that this health service would hinder business and not help it, a complete contrast to the views expressed in the Asian shop.

The effectiveness of such a project in getting men engaged with orthodox health services is difficult to estimate unless you can get good feedback from local GPs about the referrals made to them. We structured the referral form to encourage feedback but fewer than five GPs responded.

A blind attempt to rigidly replicate any tailored and targeted service will probably fail because the effectiveness of these projects is dependent on how well adapted they are to their specific situations. Ultimately, the key to success when setting up any community based health initiative targeted at a particular ethnic group is to firstly find out what that community needs and wants. Is it simply a question of providing more easily accessible and user-friendly health services or is there a deeper reluctance to acknowledge and discuss certain health problems which may be difficult to overcome with a short-term project?

SUMMARY

Aims	To reduce health inequalities.
	To tackle barriers to accessing services by taking services directly to the target community.
Where should I run sessions?	A non-healthcare setting, located within the target community and open at times when the target group will be able to attend.
	A male dominated/male friendly setting.

Where should I run sessions? (*cont.*)	An informal but confidential setting (though compromising on privacy and confidentiality may be unavoidable – a setting which offers complete privacy is no use if you can't get anyone into it).
When should I run the sessions?	At times when the men will be able and willing to access them – whilst daytime sessions will be most convenient for some, others will only be able to attend in the evenings.
	Basing a service in an establishment which is already well-attended by your target audience will increase the chances that the people that you want to reach will be there when you are.
How should I market the work?	Finding out about your target audience is essential.
	If you need to entice service users to a venue which they wouldn't ordinarily attend anyway you could try offering free food, drink and transport.
Why do men access this service?	It's free.
	Fear of rejection from the GP.
	Embarrassment about taking what they perceive to be a trivial problem to the GP.
	Having poorly-defined symptoms with which they feel unwilling to visit the doctor.
	Lack of understanding of the UK health system.
	The service is convenient – little or no effort is required to make use of it.
	The service is delivered by people with credibility in the community.
What should be included in a typical session?	This will depend on the specific nature of the service that you wish to provide and the needs of your specific target group.
	Devising a standard format will enable you to make the most efficient use of what may only be a short time with each individual and will also help potential customers to know what they can and can't expect to receive.
	Try to utilise health resources which will be best suited to the environment.
	Flexibility in the planning stage is key to devising a service which will be workable in the chosen setting.
How easy is it to replicate this type of project?	The effectiveness of this type of project is dependent on how well adapted it is to its specific situation.
	The key to success is to firstly find out what the target community needs and wants.
	In some situations it may simply be a question of providing more easily accessible, tailored and user-friendly health services; in others there may be a deeper reluctance to acknowledge and discuss certain health problems which could be difficult to overcome.

APPENDIX 9.1 CASE STUDY – 'THE MAN FROM ABROAD' (WHITE & CASH 2005)

One regular user of the service was from Islamabad and was visiting his family in England; he spoke little English and had type II diabetes which was controlled by tablets. In England he couldn't afford the tablets and felt unable to register with a GP to get a prescription. He came into contact with the HoM workers when he came in for a haircut and had the routine check that they gave. He had a high blood sugar level and came in routinely afterwards to have it monitored. He was returning to Pakistan after a few weeks. The situation of this man raises several issues:

❱ His blood sugar was high enough to cause acute problems (it was in the high twenties) when the first measurement was taken.

❱ It was difficult to interview him in depth because there was a suspicion that, because he was a visitor, there might be certain repercussions if he went to more orthodox health facilities.

❱ The need for monitoring was the result of his being unable to afford the medication that he needed and to access orthodox health services.

There is a political and moral dimension to this case. The man was accessing health services in a situation where it would have been difficult to refuse health care because to do so would have compromised the work in the barber shop. If questions were asked about the legal status of the man then the workers could reasonably expect that the uptake of the service would be seriously jeopardised.

APPENDIX 9.2 CASE STUDY – 'MY GP IS NOT INTERESTED' (WHITE & CASH 2005)

Another service user was a local shopkeeper with young children. The man was worried about his weight and the possibility that it could lead to him developing heart problems in the future. He had been made aware of the risks of being overweight after having his BMI and BP checked by the HoM workers. He had been referred to his GP but had come back to the barber shop for regular monitoring. He felt that the GP did not consider his case as important, that he didn't think that he was interested, that he was too busy to worry about such cases and would consider them as trivial. The man was clearly concerned about his weight and attended the barber shop regularly. He came for regular weight and BP checks and advice on his diet:

❱ The man felt that reducing weight was not seen as important by the GP (no matter whether the GP thought this or not).

❱ He made use of a local and convenient service. The barber shop was within walking distance of his shop.

The 'men only' nature of the barber shop meant that he was relatively comfortable having his weight and BP checked and discussing issues such as diet in public. The issue of who is watching is important and in this sense the barber shop was self-selecting – if someone was uncomfortable with the public arena then they could refuse or even go to another shop.

CHAPTER 10

Sex and relationships education in schools with boys

DENNIS JONES

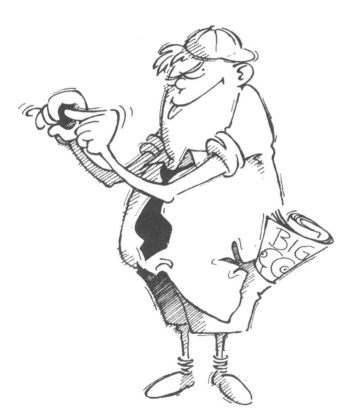

INTRODUCTION

The impetus to address the need of boys for sex education came in part from a change in the way that Bradford organised its school education system following the reorganisation of schools in the local education authority (LEA) in September 1999. Schools changed from primary schools for pupils aged 5–7, middle schools for pupils aged 8–13 and upper schools for pupils from 14–16 to a two tier system comprising only primary and upper schools. Teachers at middle schools were faced with a choice as to whether they went 'up' into secondary teaching or 'down' into primary and for many this posed a difficult choice.

With the amalgamation of the three tier system into two, however, many primary schools found themselves with boys up to the age of 11, fast approaching puberty. This change meant that primary schools now had to address sex and relationship education (SRE) for boys and girls aged up to 10. For schools that recruited middle school teachers used to teaching sex education the change was less severe, and of course it posed less of a problem with the girls as they had always had the school nurse come along and talk about menstruation. For those that had an influx of pre-pubescent boys but no middle school teachers competent in sex education the situation became fraught. In many schools the boys had largely been ignored as they had apparently had no interest in or use for information about sex.

By chance, there happened to be three male health visitors in Bradford at the time (males were outnumbered approximately 30 times by female health visitors) who were in a prime position to deliver puberty talks to the boys. One of these health visitors recruited the HoM worker as a specialist in sexual health to help him deliver these sessions, explaining that he had been called to a school where, as usual, the school nurse was giving the 'Tampax talk' to the girls while the boys were sent litter picking!

The task was to invent ways of engaging boys in a subject that seemed to both compel and repulse them in equal measure. Using games was an obvious strategy with young men because they seemed naturally to play around regardless of what type of lesson had been planned anyway.

The main thing which was learned from these initial sessions was that there needed to be some lessening of control if the lesson was to succeed, because there had to be interaction with the boys to make it work. The reason for this was that the information which they were being given wasn't value free: it was personal and likely to be different for each boy – they had to be able to talk to the worker and each other in order to discover what myths, half-truths and lies they had already been told. In addition, the words they were using were already in the language as swear words and as such forbidden in the classroom. English may not be alone in proscribing the use of sexual body part terms in polite settings, but it does seem to do so with a particular intensity that pushes them into a cauldron of repressed hysteria just waiting to bubble over. It's hardly surprising that teachers are so keen to avoid anything that stokes the fire.

AIMS

OK, that all seems clear but what do we actually do in the classroom? What are the activities for? To convey facts so that boys can be more informed about sexual information, such as how the different forms of contraception work? Or is it so that they will behave in a considerate way with their sexual partners? Or is it to help them avoid getting girls pregnant, giving their partners diseases or getting diseases themselves? Well, probably all of these; the following definition of sexual health encompasses all these questions, but it is the third element which presents the real challenge for sexual health educators:

Sexual health –

> the absence and avoidance of STIs and disorders that affect reproduction
> control of fertility and avoidance of unwanted pregnancy
> the ability to express oneself sexually gaining enjoyment and fulfilment without exploitation, oppression or abuse.

Research which examined the attitudes of excluded young men attending a youth offending team towards sex and sexual partners showed that whilst they had an understanding of the use of contraception, how condoms prevented disease and where to get hold of them, they just didn't use them. Instead they relied on a form of magical thinking which allowed them to distinguish between 'dirty girls' who where going to give them a 'dose' of something and those from whom they wouldn't catch anything.

It may be that on occasions boys need to be just given the information about how to protect themselves in order to do so, but for most you need to address:

> their attitudes to themselves and their partners
> their perceptions of what is acceptable to the male group to which they belong, and its influence on them
> their ability to change their behaviour in the light of these two factors.

These points are in line with the Government's guidance on sex and relationship education (DfEE 2000).

☞ INFO

The primary aim of the HoM sessions was to inform the boys about the changes which they were soon to experience.

The boys' primary aim was to shout out words like 'blow job' and 'tits' at every available opportunity.

HOW SHOULD I DEAL WITH COLOURFUL LANGUAGE?

This is one of the primary challenges facing someone working with young men on sex education. If you don't bring it up, they will. Most boys know perfectly well *which* the words are that they shouldn't be using but few have any idea what they really mean, other than that adults find them offensive. Hence the situation whereby they just shout them out singly and at random – it's as though each word is a trophy to hurl into the arena signifying the triumph of having merely spoken it out loud.

Our sessions on testicular self-examination (TSE) regularly began with asking the boys to call out synonyms for the terms penis and testicles. This lesson was most often held with Year 10 boys, who are more mature and less likely to fall into hysteria; even so, they often experienced anxiety which was evidenced by either embarrassed silence or calling out words accompanied by swaggering and bravado.

The Big Book of Filth (Green 1999) offers easy access to a vast cornucopia of sexual slang. Here are some favourite alternatives for the word penis:

dillywhacker	1920s United States
love truncheon	1990s
lance	late sixteenth century to early seventeenth century
quimstake	seventeenth century
pillicock	early fourteenth century to early eighteenth century – from which we get the word pillock – so just remember next time you call someone a pillock what it really means
pork sword	
beef bayonet	
love pump	
goober	(peanut) 1920s United States
Hampton	rhyming slang short for Hampton Wick – dick
flapdoodle	seventeenth century
Pecker	first brought to my attention in the novel *Slaughterhouse 5* by American author Kurt Vonnegut (1991)

Using this book illustrates to the boys:
) the huge number of words available (851 words for penis and 955 for vagina alone, the book claims) which can of course go two ways – either filling them with awe at the fertility of the human mind or despair when faced with their own meagre efforts
) that they are in the company of many others
) the variety of ways in which the sexual organs can be described.

☆ HANDY HINT

Men and boys often display this curious dichotomy – using slang much of the time in groups they feel safe in, but reluctant to use even the 'proper' terms in front of 'professionals'.

Lists of words produced by the boys can be used to discuss the use of slang in different settings, appropriate use, why some words are so offensive, who controls the language, why there are no male equivalents for the term 'slag' and so on.

In the TSE sessions, the boys then watch a video called *Know Your Balls – Check Them Out* (The Orchid Cancer Appeal 2002) in which various sports figures who have had testicular cancer speak about their experiences. When asked what was the hardest part about discussing the problem, Chris Horsman (who plays rugby for Bath) said: *'Saying the word testicle in front of the doctor'.*

The core aim of the HoM project was to get men to access health services more – if the use of language is just one of the many barriers to access then this exercise is a valuable one if it gets boys to think about the implications of their values.

WHAT DO I DO ABOUT LAUGHTER?

When standing in front of a group of boys in a classroom, having just been introduced as someone who is going to discuss sex/puberty with them, you'll probably be able to see the class seething with barely repressed laughter.

The best tactic is to offer them a minute to laugh as much as they like at the start of the session. The explosion of laughter will be loud and cathartic but will rarely last even a minute. Having got it out of the way there should be a much better level of concentration.

⚠ WARNING

If you simply ignore the boys' obvious desire to laugh, then you should expect trouble.

HOW SHOULD I DEAL WITH ANONYMOUS QUESTIONS?

By offering an opportunity to ask questions privately in a public arena you allow boys to ask about things that matter to them, whilst at the same time allowing you to address those who may be shy of asking or didn't realise that they could ask questions like that (*see* Box 10.1).

Walker and Kushner (1997) describe how young men split their worlds into the public and private:

> Boys must appear to be 'knowing', so they cannot admit ignorance or weakness. They view an adult male as someone 'who no longer needs help from anybody'. A group of 14-year-olds said that when faced with a problem, 'you bottle it up and hope it goes away'.

It seems that, faced with these dilemmas, boys do two things simultaneously: they work to build a public self (or selves) and they work to build a private self.
(pp 6–7)

Of course, you will get stupid or offensive questions, or those designed to lead you into traps: 'What does spunk taste like?'. The young man who frames this question sees himself as Machiavelli, using a clever lawyer's device designed to cast you into the depths of unimaginable humiliation in front of the group. If you are well-practised and prepared you will sidestep the question with the ease of a Premier League footballer. *'As with most of our body fluids, which are one third as salty as sea water, it's based on our evolution from the sea so it's supposed to taste salty, but I wouldn't want to put it on my chips.'* will deflect the question and demonstrate your ability to trade in salacious humour.

⚠ WARNING

Relying on ground rules e.g. 'we agreed not to talk about personal issues' could lead you into a trap. Saying something is 'personal' is more or less admitting that you've had semen in your mouth but just don't want to describe the taste. This may temporarily silence your questioner but in the process you'll also lose some valuable credibility.

Of course, it's acceptable to refer to the ground rules if you don't want to make polite conversation about times you've had semen in your mouth; this is the sort of occasion that the ground rules (or working agreements or whatever you call them) are intended for. The situation is worth reflecting on, however, because you are taking a role of *some* sort whenever you stand in front of a group of lads and whatever you do has an effect. The ground rules, like any other instrument of teaching you employ, can be used diplomatically or like a cosh.

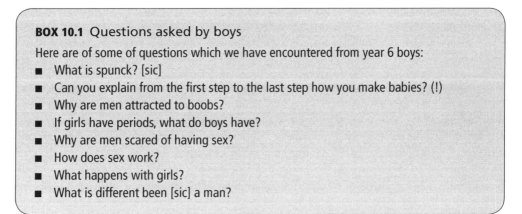

BOX 10.1 Questions asked by boys

Here are of some of questions which we have encountered from year 6 boys:

- What is spunck? [sic]
- Can you explain from the first step to the last step how you make babies? (!)
- Why are men attracted to boobs?
- If girls have periods, what do boys have?
- Why are men scared of having sex?
- How does sex work?
- What happens with girls?
- What is different been [sic] a man?

- Does sex smell?
- How do you attract girls with spots?
- Why are women sick when they are pregnant?
- Why do wimmin [sic] grow biger and biger [sic] and then shrink?
- How do breasts grow from small to big?
- What do girls start to think about?

What answers would you give to these questions?

SHOULD I GIVE PERSONAL INFORMATION?

Giving personal information is of course possible but must be done in such a way that indicates your understanding of the dilemmas faced by young men without being personal. For example, when discussing getting off a bus with an erection (an event that can be a near-death experience for a teenage boy, who must employ state of the art deception tactics or the abilities of a stage hypnotist to get himself past the thousands of pairs of eyes all fixed on his bulging trousers) you can start with such phrases as: 'You know what it's like when you're sitting on a bus and you get a 'stiffy' . . . This suggests shared experience without necessarily tagging it as personal disclosure. It may be that not all of the boys will have had the experience, but it's fairly certain that a number of them will, and by speaking to the group you can stake a claim for mutual sympathy by appealing to common experience.

Again, we are talking about making a judgement call: if you are going to appeal to common experience you have to be fairly certain that the majority of boys are going to have had that experience and can internally sigh with relief that what they thought was a perversion is actually shared by most of their peers. Saying 'You know how it is when you start trying on your mum's clothes . . .' is going to lead to frozen silence and the strong possibility of the disintegration of the lesson. There are things lads will talk about between themselves and others that they won't, although they may practise them privately. You need to know what is acceptable to talk about and what isn't.

HOW SHOULD I HANDLE RITUALISED BANTER?

Banter happens all the time between boys when they are allowed free discussion and behaviour. It's a way of establishing pecking orders, a kind of substitute for play fighting. You have to realise that if you put yourself forward as someone who wants to interact with them, you will be tested in the public arena. Are you the sort that gets easily mortified?

There are a variety of ways of dealing with banter but what is not good is to be embarrassed by it: you can join in or you can disregard it with attitude, or demonstrate a wider knowledge than they have, thereby placing them in a one-down situation. However putting the young man down in this process is also not acceptable – shaming will only create enmity.

☆ HANDY HINT

Speak to the private side of the lads – they'll be behaving in their public personas because they're together in a group but they'll still be listening from their private selves.

One of our sessions involved my teaching a group of about six boys at a pupil referral unit, accompanied by a male health visitor, talking about puberty and body changes. As well as the two health workers and the boys there were also four teachers standing apart, arms folded, holding the boys under close surveillance. Every so often they would bark instructions to the boys and at intervals this would increase in intensity and they would then remove a boy from the room. Occasionally boys would come back, but one by one they were removed from the classroom until only two remained and all the teachers had disappeared with the other boys. It was hard to see what the boys were doing wrong, as their behaviour seemed completely inoffensive, and it could only be assumed that they were giving off barely distinguishable signals which the teachers read as the beginnings of some catastrophic behaviour.

The two remaining boys were seated side by side with their chairs tilted back at the same angle. There were no teachers in the room and the boys seemed to be asking genuine questions about sex and relationships which were answered with genuine sincerity and openness. The boys started rocking on their chairs together, arriving at a perfect synchronisation, and were completely wrapped up in the discussion. It became apparent that their concentration on the dialogue and their ease with each other and the workers during the conversation was being revealed through their movement. Once you realise this, it's possible to watch for these movements as a way of gauging the level of involvement of boys – rather than seeing it as disruptive or distracted behaviour.

☆ HANDY HINT

You can often tell if boys are interested by watching for synchronisation of movement. Body language books talk about how people who are becoming interested in each other or in harmony or empathy adopt the same postures e.g. crossing the same leg, holding their heads at the same angle etc. This is the same principle, but related to movement.

This illustrates an important point from Walker and Kushner's (1997) work:

> And it may be that it is in the tension between the two [public and private selves], where the barriers come into being and crossovers occur, that attitudes and self-knowledge are formed. It is in crossing and re-crossing the space between public experimentation and private reflection, in the internal dialogue they engage in to deal with the fluidity and ambiguities they encounter, that they theorise about themselves in the world. Because it is unspoken and yet constant, this liminal self-work is difficult for the young person to explain (p.7)

> That's when I started to build the jokey, laughy, get into a bit of trouble, he-smokes-the-odd-joint, kind of thing, you know? . . . That's really when I found the identity of a young person I suppose. It was negative and non-productive in certain ways, but it was very productive in getting a feeling of self, I think. (p.10)

This should be a central goal of work in schools with boys – to help them build identities that they feel comfortable with. Of course, your contribution as a health educator is but a small influence but what you can offer is a reflection on the practical realities that a boy faces growing up. It does help if you've been a boy but this *does not prevent* females from doing the work – it may be that they just have to research the topic a bit more by asking about the experiences of puberty of their male family and friends.

HOW DOES THE WORK FIT IN WITH THE SCHOOL CURRICULUM?

> Traditionally the focus has been on girls. Boys may have felt that sex education is not relevant to them and are unable or too embarrassed to ask questions about relationships or sex. Boys are also less likely to talk to their parents about sex and relationships. For these reasons, programmes should focus on boys as much as girls at primary level as well as secondary.

> Teachers will need to plan a variety of activities which will help to engage boys as well as girls, matching their different learning styles. Single sex groups may be particularly important for pupils who come from cultures where it is only acceptable to speak about the body in single gender groups. (DfEE 2000)

The National Curriculum in England requires teachers to discuss reproduction in Key Stage 3 Science in the following areas:

❯ about the physical and emotional changes that take place during adolescence
❯ about the human reproductive system, including the menstrual cycle and fertilisation
❯ how the foetus develops in the uterus, including the role of the placenta.

So in most schools you should feel confident that the boys have at least covered the basics of biology – this may not always be the case, so it's probably best if you check it out with the teacher or the head of PSHE (personal, social and health education).

This is good practice, along with asking to see the school's sex education policy, which all schools should have:

> All schools must have an up-to-date sex and relationship education policy, drawn up by the governing body, and available to parents and for inspection.
>
> This should be developed in consultation with parents and the wider community.
>
> Primary schools should have clear parameters on what children will be taught in the transition year before moving to secondary school, and that parents be consulted.
>
> Secondary schools' policies must include how they will teach the relevant National Curriculum Science topics and how they will provide sex and relationship education as part of PSHE. (DfEE 2000)

Collaboration

Not all schools will have a sex education policy; this was certainly so in Bradford before the work of Education Bradford's PSHE advisors, who supported HoM's programme of sex education in schools. Much of their early work was getting schools to fulfil their statutory duties and write a sex and relationships education policy; they were also invaluable in organising training for teachers, learning mentors and other school staff, through which the HoM team could offer the fruits of what they had learned working with boys in school settings.

The PSHE curriculum offers the opportunity to create a planned programme of teaching and activities focussing on the emotional development of boys. Of course, it's the physical side of sex that overtly attracts boys and which they raise in the classroom. The public side of their personalities dictates that they should show maximum interest in how to 'do' heterosexual sex. Whether this type of sex is ultimately going to be the one that they prefer is not really available for discussion in the classroom; it would be a brave or very secure boy who tried to seriously discuss other forms of sexuality in an all male group. Most boys will feel much less confident inside and what might help to address that is the stuff of PSHE.

✆ WARNING

You'll need to spend some time thinking about your own sexual experiences. Talking about sex and sexual development will bring them up for you and if you haven't really examined them or your attitudes to them you may find yourself suddenly confronted by feelings that can be difficult to manage – especially in front of a group of young men.

Although many teachers might disagree, talking about biology, fertilisation, even how sex happens etc. can be relatively simple. Of course, it can be quite like running between two lines of people all throwing stones at you – at least all you have to do is run and sooner or later you'll get to the end. One classroom assistant in a primary school, who was a retired male, said to me at the end of a lesson that he thought I had 'nerves of steel', but actually I'd just delivered a rather standard lesson using a video and worksheets and allowing the boys to ask anonymous questions which were pleasant and unexceptional. It really is a question of conditioning yourself to using sexual terminology and getting used to the material.

CAN IT BE DONE?

It isn't easy to do work on sex and relationships with boys for all of the above reasons, but it is possible and it is rewarding.

The keys are:

❯ to be flexible
❯ have a sense of humour
❯ spend time practising not being embarrassed
❯ choose lessons that are fairly activity driven and maybe even competitive – use games and quizzes
❯ make sure that both you and they know what the rules are – set ground rules or working agreements. Of course the boys will challenge them, that's what rules are for isn't it?

Most boys have an innate sense of justice and when this is mobilised they will see the point of helping you maintain the rules. Give them the responsibility of helping, make it obvious: tear off the strips of paper the rules are written on and hand them out to the lads you think command the most respect.

And most of all it can be real fun!

SUMMARY

Aims	To promote sexual health among boys/young men, including: 'The ability to express oneself sexually gaining enjoyment and fulfilment without exploitation, oppression or abuse.'
	In most cases, you'll need to address their attitudes to themselves and their partners, their perceptions of what is acceptable to the male group to which they belong and its influence on them, and their ability to change their behaviour.

How should I deal with colourful language?	If you don't bring it up, they will. If you get the boys to produce a list of words this can be used to discuss the use of slang in different settings, appropriate use, why some words are so offensive, who controls the language etc. Boys will often use slang in groups they feel safe in, whilst being reluctant to use even the 'proper' terms in front of 'professionals'.
What do I do about laughter?	The best tactic is to offer the class a minute to laugh as much as they like at the start of the session. The explosion of laughter will be loud and cathartic but will rarely last even a minute. Ignoring the boys' urge to laugh will guarantee trouble.
How should I deal with anonymous questions?	Offering an opportunity to ask anonymous questions allows boys to ask about things that matter to them without embarrassment. Practice ways of deflecting stupid or offensive questions, or ones designed to lead you into traps. It's OK to refer to the ground rules but be wary of leading yourself into a trap if you rely too much on this tactic.
Should I give personal information?	Giving personal information is of course possible but must be done in such a way that indicates your understanding of the dilemmas faced by young men, without being personal. If you are going to appeal to common experience you have to be fairly certain that the majority of boys are going to have had that experience. You need to know what is acceptable to talk about and what isn't.
How should I handle ritualised banter?	Banter is a natural way of establishing pecking order. If you put yourself forward as someone who wants to interact with the boys, you will be tested in the public arena. You can join in or you can disregard it with attitude, or demonstrate a wider knowledge. Don't put the boys down. Don't get embarrassed.
How does the work fit in with the school curriculum?	In most schools you can feel confident that the boys have at least covered the basics of biology but it's best to check this with the teacher or the head of PSHE. Ask to see the school's sex education policy, which all schools should have. Spend some time thinking about your own sexual experiences – talking about sex and sexual development with others is sure to bring them up in your mind. Talking about sex, biology, fertilisation etc. can be relatively simple. It's really a question of conditioning yourself to using sexual terminology and getting used to the material.
Can it be done?	It isn't easy but it can be done. Have a sense of humour and practise not being embarrassed about the material. Make your lessons activity driven. Be flexible but set clear ground rules.

CHAPTER 11

Anti-bullying work

MERV PEMBERTON

INTRODUCTION

The HoM anti-bullying work began when the Airedale team were asked by health visitors in Scarborough if they did any work around bullying and young men. One of the HoM workers had personal experience of being bullied at school and this provided an additional motivation to set up an anti-bullying programme, with support from a youth worker who was working with us at the time.

We work with both genders for the simple reason that it's become much more common for boys to socialise with girls. At one time boys wouldn't really hang around with girls because they would be teased, but nowadays you see a lot more boys walking round with girls and feeling comfortable with it. Because they're regularly mixing with each other, it would be ineffective to try to tackle bullying by targeting boys and girls separately. Additionally, many boys' best friends are now girls, and if there's a problem for the boy it will often be his female friends, rather than the boy himself, who will talk about it. Often it's girls who encourage the boys to tell the truth and address an issue.

☆ HANDY HINT

When working with girls as well as boys it's naturally much better to refer to yourself as an anti-bullying worker, rather than a men's health worker.

Most of the anti-bullying sessions take place in primary schools but a lot of the work is also done in the community, working with youth groups and trying to get youth workers to see what bullying is and how it can occur. Youth workers have children and young men coming through their doors wanting to talk about feelings of being bullied, either in the community or at work, and we're there to try to support them as best we can.

AIMS

The aims of the work are to get people to recognise, and also to feel comfortable with reporting, whatever *they* feel is bullying. Successfully putting across the anti-bullying message depends on having third party involvement, rather than someone who's directly involved with the school, community centre or whatever the setting may be.

Getting the message across requires addressing the different age groups specifically. With children in Key Stage 1 or Reception we use the theme of *Sharing and Caring* rather than referring to bullying, because the term 'bullying' isn't always something which they understand. They're at the age where they're learning to share and care, and it's introduced in that way, rather than by saying 'we're doing anti-bullying work', because that just goes over young children's heads. The idea is to catch bullying early and get children to recognise that it's not right to push somebody in the playground, or to push in, or just because somebody else has something to take it off them. We hope as they grow older they'll learn to carry that message through the rest of their lives.

With Key Stage 2 pupils the aim is to get them to understand what bullying is – what the bully does, and the effect of being part of a group which is encouraging someone else to bully.

WHERE SHOULD I RUN SESSIONS?

Most of this kind of work will take place in schools, but you may be asked to run sessions in community centres, with groups in the community, or even in a prison. We've had people from the church and the mosque ask us to go in and do some work because they feel that they get quite a bit of bullying in there. You might think that in a church or a mosque you wouldn't have bullying because it's a place of worship, but it does still go on there. We are also asked to work with Scouts, Brownies and Guides, and at all sorts of places where you wouldn't think bullying would happen much. Another aspect of anti-bullying work is working with people with learning difficulties so that they recognise when somebody is bullying them. Bullying, of course, comes in all forms and it's always important to explain that it's not simply about using physical violence.

WHEN SHOULD I RUN SESSIONS?

It's really never too soon to begin anti-bullying work with young people, so we do sessions in primary schools first and then come back and do transitional work with pupils when they're moving school. When children are about to go up into upper school they hear rumours going round that they'll have their heads put down the toilet etc., and we try to get them to realise that whilst this could happen, and might happen, it shouldn't be accepted as inevitable. One of the things we do in the transitional sessions is to make children aware of potential problems, for example, that if you cycle now to your middle school or primary school it's quite safe to go and check your bike at break time without being picked on, but when you're at upper school it will be best not to go and check your bike all the time because you're likely then to become a potential target for bullies.

In the upper schools we like to see children when they come into Year 7, then in Year 8, and that's normally enough to steer the ship.

Sometimes we get a cry for help from a school when they have a big problem or a crisis, but that's often not the right time to do anti-bullying work because the crisis has already happened and trying to resolve it doesn't always help.

HOW SHOULD I MARKET THE WORK?

Teacher 'away days' can offer a good opportunity to give a talk presenting your work. Once your service becomes known about you'll find that schools come to you as teachers tell each other about the service. Getting your work covered in the press also helps to raise awareness.

We usually wait to be invited into a school rather than asking if we can do a session, unless it's as a result of the health needs assessment when we can say: 'There's x percentage of bullying going on in this school – can we have a look at it and see how we can change this?'.

⊛ WARNING

Be careful to plan ahead and not let the schools all leave anti-bullying sessions until the end of the year when the children are starting to get restless. Getting the sessions incorporated into the citizenship classes makes it easier to spread them out over the year.

Teachers generally welcome the idea of having the sessions because the anti-bullying message can come over better from a visitor, rather than from a teacher who's in the school full time. Pupils get close to teachers whether they like them or not, and sometimes teachers lose the respect required to talk convincingly on this kind of subject. A lot of bullying is actually by the pupils toward the teachers. Sometimes pupils will be open and put their hands up when asked if they think that they've bullied their teachers or their parents.

☆ HANDY HINT

If you can get members of the sixth form trained to act as mentors or peer support for Year 7s this will ensure that there are people around to support them all the way through the year.

WHY DO PEOPLE USE THE SERVICE?

Most of the schools we're working with have put anti-bullying into the school curriculum so the session is one of the pupils' lessons in citizenship. The Office for Standards in Education (Ofsted) like this service because they know that the school is getting someone in to address the issue. Having the sessions as normal lessons provides a captive audience. When working in community centres and community areas obviously it's voluntary whether participants stay or don't.

☆ HANDY HINT

Don't forget that bullying doesn't always happen in school. It can happen on the way home from school or the way in and sometimes comes from pupils from another school who are passed on the way.

If you look around at the audience while giving the talk you can see from their facial reactions that some are thinking 'That's me, that's what I'm doing'. Often these people will come up to you at the end and admit that bullying is what they're doing to their friends or other people, and ask how they can change. Of course some will come and say 'Well, that's me but I don't want to change'.

From the young people's perspective, the service provides somebody totally different to talk to and some use it just to see what knowledge they can take away from it. Sometimes they're worried about friends who aren't telling people the truth – aren't telling their parents or their teachers what's happening to them.

WHAT'S THE STRUCTURE OF THE SESSIONS?

The structure changes depending on the age group and the agenda you've gone in with at the time. For example, there may be homophobic bullying which needs to be addressed, or you may be talking to people with learning difficulties. It's important to keep in mind who you're talking to, the level at which you can pitch your talk and where you are.

At Key Stage 1 and Key Stage 2 we begin by showing children a red and green apple, ask them what these are, then ask them what colour they are, cut them in half, ask about the size, the colour of the apples and the insides of the apples – which are the same. This is to show that that's how we are as people – maybe different on the outside, but all the same on the inside. Then we use role plays to address different themes, such as boys and girls sharing toys, playing together, and sharing in achievements, e.g. if somebody receives a certificate, it's not only for them but for the whole class and school. In Key Stage 2 we bring in themes such as fashion, treating people differently (e.g. for achieving, or for wearing glasses), and using mobile phones and text messages. With Years 7–11 we then move up to the full Powerpoint presentation, an outline of which is included at the end of the chapter.

The structure will always be flexible anyway because people will ask questions about different things, not necessarily towards the end. If you realise something's a bit sensitive and somebody's getting a bit upset you can steer the discussion away and then ask that person, or a small group if they've got friends with them, to come and see you at the end of the lesson. Nine out of ten times it will be somebody in the same class who is bullying them, so it doesn't help if you bring the subject into the light there and then.

What you will tend to find is that those pupils in the lower attainment groups will lose concentration if you do the Powerpoint presentation all in one session, so it works better to do half of it and then stay for the rest of the lesson and talk with the children about general things – the community, what's going on in their lives and your work. Then, after they've had a break of about two weeks, go in and do the other half of the lesson with them. This seems to work really well because when we go back in for the second half there will be people reminding us of what we talked about a couple of weeks before, when normally they would have forgotten what they did in their lessons a couple of weeks previously. We also get reports from pupils and teachers saying how different their behaviour has been since the first session, so it's obvious that they have been interested in the lesson.

HOW LONG SHOULD THE SESSIONS BE?

The talks last an hour in total but it's important not to disappear straight afterwards as you'll want to be around in case anyone has any questions or wants to talk. We say that we'll be there at the end or maybe in the Year Head's room, or if they don't catch us then we'll be back in school on a certain date to do a further session. Often in the meantime we'll receive an email from the teacher listing who wants to meet for a talk. Schools tend to be quite lenient in that they'll let you have half a lesson or whatever you need to meet a child who wants to see you. Sometimes children will want to talk with their parents and the teacher present, but either way it's important to always have a chaperone when the children come to see you, whether it's a teacher, a parent or one of your colleagues.

☸ WARNING

Some children make up stories just to get somebody into trouble. Always try to read between the lines and think 'Does this sound right; is this the full picture?'

When someone comes up at the end and tells you about something that's happened, the first thing is to find out whether or not they've spoken to anybody about it. If they've told nobody then you should tell them that they need to see a teacher about it. Sometimes the person they want to talk to might not be their own teacher, it's just a question of finding somebody that they feel comfortable with. Offer to come with them to provide support if they want it and be sure to emphasise the importance of telling the truth.

WHAT SKILLS AND EXPERIENCE DO I NEED?

With Key Stage 1, role plays are the main method for putting the message across, so a willingness and ability to effectively deliver these, as well as the Powerpoint presentations used at Key Stage 2 and above, is obviously an essential requirement. There's no reason, however, why someone would need to be a youth worker or already be working with people in order to do the work.

The main thing is to have an awareness of young people and how they're interacting with each other, so that you know what the issues are at any time and can keep your presentations relevant. For example, at the time of writing, there are a lot more girls than boys bullying, for whatever reason. Also there's recently been a lot of text bullying going on, but this is now beginning to drift out and be replaced by instant messenger bullying at evenings, weekends and holidays, over the Internet. We tell teachers that they'll find that on Monday morning or after a holiday there'll be a lot of trouble because children have been at home but in contact through MSN, and tensions have built up which explode when they're back in school together.

Keeping an ear to the ground is therefore very important. A good technique is to go to McDonald's on a Saturday, or to the bus station or train station, where there will be a lot of young people hanging around, and just watch how they're interacting with each other. Another tip is to contact schools and ask if you can do playground duties, just to be aware of things and see what's going on.

☻ WARNING

This isn't really a job for the faint-hearted! It isn't unknown to have 25 kids running at you at once shouting: 'It's that bully man; let's bully him!' and taking you off your feet!

WHAT EQUIPMENT DO I NEED?

When doing role plays with the *Caring and Sharing* work in Key Stage 1 you'll need a few props. We used to use a scooter and a little trike, but the trike was falling to bits, so for health and safety reasons we had to give that up. In one of the role plays we did, one HoM worker would get on the trike and another on the scooter. The worker on the trike would then bump into the one on the scooter:

'You're not my friend.

Why? We've always been friends.

Well what's that scooter?

My grandma bought it for my birthday.

Well you're not gonna go around with me unless you get a trike!'

We also use Barbie and Action Man to show that boys are allowed to play with dolls – that Action Man and Max Steel are just male dolls (although you can get funny looks walking through a school with Barbie sticking out of your back pocket!). Sometimes we consider fashion, for example not leaving out new kids who don't have a uniform because they may have just moved to the area and their parents may not be able to afford to buy them one at that moment. Basically, the idea is to use props with the role plays to try and make the lesson as visual as possible.

SUMMARY

Aims	To get people to recognise, and also to feel comfortable in reporting, whatever they consider to be bullying.
	With children at Key Stage 1 or Reception we use the theme of *Sharing and Caring* rather than referring to bullying.
	With Key Stage 2 the aim is to get children to understand what 'bullying' is.
Where should I run sessions?	Mostly this kind of work will take place in schools, but you may be asked to run sessions in a wide variety of community groups and settings.
When should I run sessions?	It's really never too soon to begin anti-bullying work with young people, so we do sessions in primary schools first and then come back and do transitional work with pupils when they're moving school.
	Sometimes we get a cry for help from a school when they have a crisis, but that's often not the right time to do anti-bullying work.
How should I market the work?	Teacher 'away days' can offer a good opportunity to present your work.
	Once your service becomes known about you'll find that schools come to you as teachers tell each other about the service.
Why do people use the service?	Most of the schools we're working with have put anti-bullying into the school curriculum. Having the session as a citizenship lesson provides a captive audience.
	From the young people's perspective the service provides somebody totally different to talk to.
What's the structure of the sessions?	The structure changes depending on the age group and the agenda you've gone in with at that time.
	The structure will always vary because you'll get people asking questions about different things, not necessarily towards the end.
	You'll find that pupils in the lower attainment groups will lose concentration if you do a full session of Powerpoint so it works better to do it in two halves.
How long should the sessions be?	The talks last an hour in total but it's important not to disappear straight afterwards in case anyone has any questions or wants to talk.
	Specify a date to return to the school to do a further session. Teachers can email you in the meantime with a list of pupils who wish to talk.
What skills and experience do I need?	An ability to effectively deliver both role plays and Powerpoint presentations is an essential requirement, as well as having the skills to talk to pupils on a one-to-one basis.
	It's very important to be able to maintain an awareness of young people's issues so as to keep up to date with changes in young people's behaviour, e.g. text and instant messenger bullying.
What equipment do I need?	When doing role plays with the *Caring and Sharing* work at Key Stage 1 you'll need a few props. Try to make sessions as visual as possible.

APPENDIX 11.1 BEAT THE BULLY!
Presentation for years 7–11

The nature of bullying

There are many definitions of bullying, but most consider it to be:

❱ deliberately hurtful (including aggression)
❱ repeated often over a period of time
❱ difficult for victims to defend themselves against.

Bullying can take many forms, but three main types are:

❱ *physical* – hitting, kicking, taking belongings
❱ *verbal* – name calling, insulting, making offensive remarks
❱ *indirect* – nasty stories being spread about someone, exclusion from social groups, being made the subject of malicious rumours.

Name calling is the most common direct form. This may be because of individual characteristics, but pupils can be called nasty names because of their ethnic origin, nationality, colour or some form of disability.

Who is involved in bullying – and where?

Both boys and girls bully others. Usually boys are bullied by boys, but girls are bullied by girls and boys. The most common perpetrators are individual boys or groups of several boys. Children who bully others can come from any kind of family, regardless of social class or cultural background.

Although bullying can occur during the journey to or from school, e.g. extortion or theft of possessions such as mobile phones, most typically it takes place in school. It is more likely where adult surveillance is intermittent. In primary schools, up to three-quarters of bullying takes place in the playground. In secondary schools it is also likely to be outdoors, but classrooms, corridors and toilets are common sites.

Usually one pupil starts bullying a victim. There are often other pupils present. These may:

❱ help the bully by joining in
❱ help bully by watching, laughing and shouting encouragement
❱ remain resolutely uninvolved
❱ help the victim directly, tell the bullies to stop, or fetch an adult.

Bullying by race, gender, sexual orientation or disability

Incidents can include:

❱ verbal abuse by name calling, racist jokes and offensive mimicry
❱ physical threats or attacks
❱ wearing of provocative badges or insignia
❱ bringing in racist leaflets, comics or magazines
❱ inciting others to behave in a racist way

❭ racist graffiti or other written insults – even against food, music, dress or customs

❭ refusing to cooperate in work or in play.

Sexual bullying

Sexual bullying impacts on both genders. Boys are also victims – of girls and other boys. A case of proven sexual assault is likely to lead to the exclusion of the perpetrator. In general, sexually bullying is characterised by:

❭ abusive name calling

❭ looks and comments about appearance, attractiveness, emerging puberty

❭ inappropriate and uninvited touching

❭ sexual innuendoes and propositions

❭ pornographic material, graffiti with sexual content

❭ in its most extreme form, sexual assault or rape.

Special groups

Pupils with special educational needs (SEN) or disabilities may not be able to articulate experiences as well as other children. However, they are often at greater risk of being bullied, both directly and indirectly and usually about their specific difficulties or disability.

Strategies include:

❭ referring to such issues in anti-bullying policies

❭ reflecting on how teachers behaviour might unintentionally trigger bullying

❭ avoiding undue attention to differences between SEN children and others

❭ making classroom activities sensitive to the needs of SEN children

❭ teaching assertiveness and other social skills

❭ peer mentoring

❭ teaching victims to say 'no' or get help

❭ role-playing in dealing with taunts

❭ providing special resource rooms at playtimes and lunchtimes.

Being bullied

If you are being bullied:

❭ try to stay calm and look as confident as you can

❭ be firm and clear – look them in the eye and tell them to stop

❭ get away from the situation as quickly as possible

❭ tell an adult what has happened straight away

after you have been bullied:

❭ tell a teacher or another adult in your school

❭ tell your family

❭ if you are scared to tell an adult by yourself, ask a friend to come with you

❭ keep speaking up until someone listens and does something to stop the bullying

> if your school has peer support service, use it
> don't blame yourself for what has happened.

When you are talking to an adult about bullying, be clear about:
> what has happened to you
> how often it has happened
> who was involved
> who saw what was happening
> where it happened
> what you have done about it already.

If you find it difficult to talk to anyone at school or at home, ring Child Line, Freephone 0800 1111, or write to them at Freepost 1111, London N1 0BR.

The phone call or letter is free. It is a confidential helpline.

Bullying and the law

> A pupil waits for another pupil after school and tells him/her that he/she is going to be beaten up.
>   – *Section 39 Assault: there is no need for physical contact for the assault to be committed.*
> A pupil takes another pupil's dinner money from them by telling them that if they don't hand it over they will be 'thumped'.
>   – *Robbery: in taking the money (theft) the person put the victim in fear of being assaulted.*
> A pupil sends another a nasty text message every night for a week.
>   – *Harassment: repeated more than once and causes harassment and alarm.*
> A pupil repeatedly calls another pupil derogatory names that relate to their skin colour.
>   – *Uses threatening/abusive/insulting words/behaviour (racially motivated). Due to it being a race hate incident the offender will receive a higher level tariff penalty.*
> A pupil deliberately pushes another pupil over causing slight injury.
>   – *Section 39 Assault: No visible injury is required.*
>   – *Section 47 Assault: A visible injury would be required to prove this offence.*
> A group of pupils go and sit outside the house of another pupil and pull faces at him or her when they appear at the window.
>   – *Harassment (possibly).*
>   – *Public Nuisance.*

CHAPTER 12

Health sessions in housing projects

MARTIN SAMANGAYA

INTRODUCTION

The HoM team have worked with various housing projects in Bradford. The majority of young people accommodated in housing projects have come from broken homes and have been in and out of care. In total, there are four housing projects in Bradford into which we have had some input. Our work with these projects began through referrals from outside agencies, requesting our input with these young people. Colleagues in Family Planning had been doing sexual health sessions at one of the housing projects with female residents and requests were made for similar services for young men. However, Family Planning colleagues were using traditional methods of teaching and as a result there was a general lack of interest from the young people.

The majority of the young people accommodated in the housing projects are in the 'hard to engage with' category and therefore a different approach was needed to get their attention, curiosity and participation. The work with three of the housing projects, namely City Centre Project, Vicar Lane and Bradford Foyer, was affected by work pressures. We had to prioritise other areas of our work and other regular commitments across the city, and it became practically impossible to sustain the work in all four housing projects. As a result, we are at present only working with one housing project in Bradford.

AIMS

This chapter describes the work taking place at one of the four housing projects with which the HoM team have been involved. This work has been going on for four years and was initiated when they heard about our work with the other housing projects in Bradford.

The project provides temporary accommodation of between six months and two years for seven young people aged 16–25 years who are homeless or at risk of being homeless. It provides a high level of support and houses some of the most difficult to place young people who may have multiple and complex needs. These may include a history of offending (some having been in prison) and substance and/or alcohol abuse. Some of these young people would have poor school attendance records and may have missed out on the Personal Health Social and Citizenship Education (PHSE) or any health related sessions at school. The project helps residents to develop life skills and social skills, to access training and education and also to have the assistance of a resettlement worker.

HOW DO YOU ENGAGE THE YOUNG MEN?

Residents must attend a health session as a condition of their contract to stay in the house. The fact that their attendance at the health session forms part of their contract makes it easier for our team to organise sessions, as we are assured of their presence. HoM have been running sessions at regular set times every month, for example, every first Thursday of the month, unless there are any events taking place in the house, which means postponing the session to a later date. We tend to announce the sessions four weeks in advance and the residents are informed so that they can be in the house at that particular time. The sessions usually last for about 40–60 minutes.

☆ HANDY HINT

An innovative and adaptable approach is needed to be successful in engaging with young people (HDA 2002).

It's also important to have a non-judgemental attitude and reassure young people about confidentiality, so that they are aware that they can share or ask anything in confidence (TPU 2000).

When the work first started at this housing project it involved sessions on sexual health, STIs and contraception. The sessions then expanded to talking about general health issues affecting the young people. A strategy was developed to involve the young people and workers at the housing project, and asking them to suggest any health related topics or issues they wanted us to address. Involving them like this means we are talking about issues that are relevant to their needs and also something that they have an interest in. Another strategy employed has involved discussing current health issues highlighted by the local or national media. In some of our work incentives, for example pens, mugs, sperm-shaped key rings (to name just a few) have often been used as a way of encouraging the young people to attend and participate in the sessions.

☣ WARNING

Major events like World Cup football matches must be considered when planning the sessions. It would be unproductive to have a session on the same day as a big England game, for example.

BOX 12.1 Case Study

It was noted by the workers that most of the residents' oral hygiene was appalling. One reason for this was because the young people had picked up from a chewing gum advert that if you chew gum regularly it is good for your teeth: they took this literally and thought that it was alright to chew gum *instead* of brushing their teeth.

A session was organised by the team, which involved liaising with the community oral health team who gave us literature and visual aids (a large model of a set of teeth and toothbrush) for demonstration purposes, as well as free toothbrushes and toothpaste. The session was kept simple and covered issues about gum disease, how to look after your teeth, the problems of not brushing regularly and registering with a dentist. Three of the residents' teeth needed immediate attention and referrals were made by the team to the Bradford Dental Service for Asylum Seekers and Homeless Clients. The clients were seen within a short space of time and their teeth treated and cleaned. After their visit to the dentist, one of the workers commented that two of the residents were so impressed and pleased with the way their teeth looked that they have started to make a lot of effort to brush their teeth regularly to keep them clean.

HOW DO YOU BUILD RAPPORT?

The turnover of residents every year or month depends on the length of time each resident needs to be accommodated. There have been residents who have been at the house for over a year; you get to know them better each month and you also start to build relationships with new residents. The work we have been doing has gone beyond doing health sessions each month and disappearing. There have been occasions when sessions have been cancelled for reasons beyond anyone's control but the team had not been informed and had turned up for the session. On such occasions, the team would stay around and use the opportunity to engage with the young people, playing pool or computer games, watching football or *The Simpsons* or simply just chatting. Through this interaction we have been able to build relationships with the residents so that they can see us as normal, ordinary 'blokes' rather than authority figures.

☆ **HANDY HINT**

Relationships built with the residents and staff over the years have made it easy for our HoM to signpost the residents to other services.

Our attire when we visit the project is informal – the sort of clothes the young people would wear themselves. We don't dress up in suits and ties, as we feel that this can create a barrier between us and the young people and they might end up perceiving us as authority figures. We believe that through the strategy of engaging as ordinary men, young people are more likely to feel at ease, relate and maybe ask us about any health worries.

BOX 12.2 Case Study

On one occasion when a session had been cancelled, our team member stayed and started chatting with the young people. One of the residents asked if he could have a word in private, he wanted to ask about certain aspects of health that had been bothering him and what he should do about them. He had a medical problem which had bothered him since he was young; he had never told anyone about it as it had never been an issue but now in his late teens he couldn't ignore it any more. He had a chat and explained what had been happening. We found out more information about his condition and possible causes, and the resident was encouraged to go and talk to his GP. The team offered to go with him to see the GP if he needed moral support.

WHAT FORM DO THE SESSIONS TAKE?

One of the things we have learned from working with residents is to be well prepared and keep things as simple as possible. There have been times when we have prepared material for 40 minutes and have ended up doing only 20 minutes, and there have also been times when we have prepared for 20–25 minutes and have carried on for 40–60 minutes. It is important to use good judgement to see how sessions are going and if there is a general lack of interest in the session to keep it short and either move onto something a bit more interesting or finish the session. There have been moments, for example, when we have been doing a session on personal hygiene and the residents want to talk about STIs instead of sticking to the prepared session. In order to avoid losing the residents' attention and interest, we have often diverted and talked about the issues they want to explore or discuss.

BOX 12.3 Case Study

One of the sessions we facilitated at the house was on food hygiene, storage and preparation. We made this session interesting by offering to cook a meal for all the residents. We spent 15 minutes at the beginning talking about basic principles of food hygiene and then went into the kitchen to cook the meal. As we were providing a free meal for the residents, they were all looking forward to the session and the food. We selected an easy and healthy meal (spaghetti bolognese) which was freshly prepared for the residents. There were about six residents on that day and in the kitchen we went through all the aspects we had discussed, including washing vegetables, handling meat and not contaminating vegetables with uncooked meat. The idea of seeing things being done practically made learning interactive for the residents. It generated interest, with everyone helping in the kitchen and we later shared a meal together and engaged a little more in an informal setting.

WHAT ARE THE KEY THINGS FOR MAKING IT WORK?
Staff motivation

Our experiences of working in the housing projects have revealed that the sessions are more likely to be a success if project staff working with the residents are motivated and supportive of the work you are doing. This might sound like common sense, but staff support and involvement is critical as they play a role in reminding the residents of the time and dates you are coming and also making sure none of the residents double book themselves on the day.

Good working partnerships

A good working partnership with other multidisciplinary team members and agencies is also vital as their input may be required for particular sessions, or you may need to refer the young people to other agencies. In our work we have used other colleagues who are specialists in certain areas to come and do sessions on a particular topic, for example, a smoking cessation advisor and a dietician.

Good reputation

As a team of men's health workers it is important to maintain a good reputation in the various work you are involved with in your local area, which means delivering your sessions and conducting yourselves in a professional manner. The way we have conducted ourselves as a team has been very important for our image because a lot of the work we have been involved with has come about from people contacting us after hearing good things about us and our work.

It's alright to say 'I don't know'

There is a temptation sometimes to be a 'jack-of-all-trades', but it is important to be true to yourself, and this means if you don't know something admitting it to the young people. Young people can sense when someone doesn't know what they are talking about and previous experience has taught us to say 'I don't know the answer but will find out the details and bring them next time'.

Try new things and take risks

In our work we have tried new things and in many cases taken risks to implement new ideas; some of our ideas have worked and some have failed. The good thing about doing this is you can always learn from your mistakes or reflect on the reasons why some of the ideas have not worked.

SUMMARY

Aims	The housing projects house some of the most difficult to place young people who may have multiple and complex needs. Some of these young people have poor school attendance records and may have missed out on the Personal Health Social and Citizenship Education (PHSE) or any health related sessions at school.
How do you engage the young men?	Residents must attend a health session as part of their contract to stay in the house.
	We tend to announce the sessions four weeks in advance and the residents are informed so that they can be in the house at that particular time.
	To make the sessions relevant we ask residents for any health issues which they wish to discuss, or talk about health issues which are in the media.
How do you build a rapport?	The work we have been doing has gone beyond doing health sessions each month and disappearing. We take opportunities to engage with the young people – playing pool, computer games, watching TV or simply chatting – so that they see us as ordinary 'blokes'.
	Our attire when we visit the project is informal – the sort of clothes the young people would wear themselves.
What form do the sessions take?	The sessions usually last for about 40–60 minutes.
	Be well prepared and keep things as simple as possible.
	Always be ready to be flexible. Use your judgement to see how sessions are going and if there is a general lack of interest move onto something a bit more interesting or finish the session.
What are the key things for making it work?	Staff motivation Good working partnership Good reputation It's alright to say 'I don't know' Try new things and take risks.

PART THREE

CHAPTER 13

A brief history of HoM – a personal perspective

DENNIS JONES

In January 1993 I decided to organise a professional development day on men's health as part of a regional training programme for health promotion officers. I thought about it for a while and rang round places to see what sort of activities there were specifically directed at men. I knew that there were some activities around that involved men getting naked and sitting in sweat lodges and crying a lot and that sort of thing, but I didn't think that this would be viewed as legitimate health promotion by my colleagues.

I was pleased with the programme that I eventually came up with. Jeff Hearn, who had written books about men and who worked at Bradford University, gave a theoretical overview of men's health and then there were workshops on men and drugs, men as carers, men living with HIV and men and driving. I thought that was a fair summary of men's health at the time. One cultural note that I must mention is that the workshop on men and driving was run by two probation officers from Nottingham who called it *Driving with Rambo*.

There was one moment that I treasured when a nurse from Hull, who had worked for quite a while on a cardiac ward, had a 'light bulb' moment: she had just realised, she said, that the vast majority of people who had been on her ward were men. It was like the business of goldfish not recognising they inhabit water because it surrounds them the whole time. I understood from that moment that a lot of the work involved in developing men's health was getting people to pay attention to what was going on around them – and that certainly included the male half of the population.

My next opportunity to think about men and their health came in 1997 when I was approached by a male health visitor – one of only three in Bradford – who wanted me to help him run a training day for his health visitor colleagues on the subject of fatherhood. In July we put on a training day for health visitors, school nurses and midwives that tried to grapple with the reasons why men seemed so often to be left out of the picture by the various services directed at children and their mothers.

The opinion offered by some of the female health visitors and midwives on the course was that men weren't really competent to look after their children, an opinion with which the mothers often colluded. These were the attitudes that my male health visitor colleague wanted to challenge:

> *The father's view of himself as an irrelevance is often reinforced by professionals such as health visitors who, even if the father is present, can quite unashamedly direct all comments to the mother, or tend to patronise fathers when they turn up at the clinic in charge of their babies.*

I had another moment of enlightenment when taking feedback from an exercise that asked the participants to reflect on their experiences with their own fathers. The anger that poured from one woman – a health visitor in her fifties – was both sad and disturbing. I thought *'No wonder this woman has no time for the men she encounters in her daily work'*.

My health visitor colleague and I began to collaborate on other projects, working in schools and developing ways to engage boys in the classroom. He came to see me one day saying that he had been contacted by a school where the girls got the familiar menstruation talk from the school nurse whilst the boys were sent litter picking (I have related this story elsewhere in the book. I relate it everywhere – I find it so extraordinary).

We were joined by the two other male health visitors who were also beginning to do puberty talks in schools and began regular meetings over the next couple of years to offer each other support. We talked of the ten per cent of health visitors' time that should be devoted to public health and how we could use it to develop support for men and their health.

It was during this time, in early 1999, that we embarked on an ambitious plan to create a mobile men's health clinic with some Health Action Zone money that had been set aside for developing men's health. We got as far as viewing a bus and having preliminary negotiations with a bodywork company regarding its conversion, before we were 'rumbled' – apparently none of us was senior enough to authorise such radical expenditure.

A further addition to the group was a worker from the local authority who was part of the Council's HIV Unit; he was the one who eventually provided the name for the project. Among his suggestions were: *SMASH!* – Supporting Men And Sexual Health; *MALE* – Men And Living, Equally; *DUDE!* – Definitely U Deserve Equality and, the one we eventually went with, HoM – *Health of Men*. It was only later and with mixed feelings that we discovered we had named our project after a brand of underwear.

Finally we were joined by a student who on qualifying took up a post in

Keighley. I say finally, although this isn't really an accurate description of the process, because HoM accreted like making a snowball – we were constantly trying to add members (and still are). The ones that stuck became part of the network and ultimately part of the HoM team.

Subsequently the final member to join the team created and applied for the position of HoM facilitator and began building a HoM team in Keighley by getting sums of money from various sources and appointing new staff. He felt his way through funding organisations and often thought 'outside the box' without being daunted by the rules and regulations.

In October 1999 this team ran a health week for the town offering information, advice, exercise demonstrations and entertainment in an attempt to attract men along to consider their health. This was the first *Men's Health Week*, which has now become a national event through the influential growth of the Men's Health Forum. This was also the year that work started on a men's health website (www. healthofmen.com), the first British based website dealing exclusively with male health issues.

To try to establish a baseline of knowledge we wrote a questionnaire that asked for respondents' opinions on where they would most prefer to be offered health advice and of what type. Out of a total of 393 respondents, 71% wanted more information – most particularly on heart disease, stress, diet and exercise. If they were worried about a health problem the majority – contrary to research – thought that they would first consult their GP, next a partner and then read up on it.

We asked a series of questions:
> Who is the healthiest man you know?
> How did he get that way?
> And why aren't all men as healthy?

The answers were not a surprise: the most frequent answer was Linford Christie, who was in the news for getting an OBE in 1998. Clearly many of the respondents felt that health equated with fitness, and Christie was one of the most high profile athletes at the time, attracting considerable press attention for his 'lunchbox' (a reference to his genitalia which were outlined by his close-fitting shorts). This was also apparently considered a sign of health.

There were several other sportsmen mentioned, their qualification for the healthiest man being that they trained and kept themselves fit. The answer to the question 'Why aren't all men as healthy?' was consistently given as lack of time and too much alcohol and smoking, indicating that most men knew what it took to be healthy but felt that it was a hard thing to achieve.

The next most healthy man came as more of a surprise, as many respondents picked their father and in one instance grandfather. A typical reason for this was: *'Looked after himself as a kid to the present day.'* This was a consistent finding and again equated health with fitness, often achieved through 'physical work' and moderation in their behaviour. Most of the men who answered the questionnaire knew that lack of moderation in eating and drinking, and smoking and not exercising were responsible for ill-health.

The results of the questionnaire set the agenda and location of the men's health drop-ins in Keighley, some of which worked and others of which didn't. The process of developing health resources for men took on more firmly the pattern that came to characterise the project as a whole, that of 'suck it and see'. We were fortunate to have a highly motivated group of workers with a wide variety of skills and lots of ideas. They reminded me in some ways of the *A-Team*: a group of eccentric individuals with divergent skills welded into an effective fighting unit – but without the cigars and jewellery. In addition we had a fair degree of freedom in deciding what kind of interventions to use. This concoction led to a number of inventive strategies to try to engage men in their own health.

We used the accepted wisdom based on the research by Lloyd of *Working with Men* and others (Lloyd, 1998; 2001): that men responded better when health advice was made easier to access by taking it to where they were and making it accessible in other ways e.g. by making it more informal. An example of this was the pub quiz, the aim of it being to provide health related information in a socially acceptable format, to raise the profile of the HoM project, to introduce men's health related topics into the social setting of a pub and to encourage the association of health and fun.

The first one we tried out in the social club of a local transport workers union, with prizes donated by local businesses. I remember two things about the evening in particular. The 'audience' was for the most part middle-aged couples who were reasonably enthusiastic about participating. The subject matter and the audience between them gave the evening the air of a *Carry On* film with a lot of joking and teasing – one of the questions asked how many times a year people in Britain had sex and another the average length of an erect penis; the differences in answers between members of the same couple were highly entertaining.

The other thing I remember was a late middle-aged man who stood at the bar drinking with his back to everyone in the room. We were reading out the answers and giving bits of information as we went along; when we came to the answers about the prostate he turned around and asked 'What's a prostate?' My colleague briefly explained and for a moment there was an interaction with a man who would not have normally talked to anyone about health issues.

One thing we learned from doing the quiz the first couple of times was that if we made all the questions 'medical' then very few people were able to answer them. We needed to intersperse them between more general knowledge questions – people like to feel that they have a reasonable chance of competing or they get demotivated. One of the times we included mostly medical questions, though, the quiz was won quite decisively by a group of young women, which I guess says something about men and their knowledge of health.

The HoM Airedale PCT team have done about ten of these quizzes now and interaction with the customers has always been a major feature of the evenings.

In venues where the team have repeated the quiz they have always had good numbers in attendance. The pub quizzes are generally newsworthy projects and therefore were good for raising the profile of the HoM project as a whole.

During this period the group was actively seeking to build networks and alliances and in Keighley this was greatly accelerated by one of the team who seemed to know most people in the town. Many connections were made with trades and workplaces: printers, building societies, shops and banks – not what NHS staff would consider to be 'the usual suspects' but places where we could find men in abundance. A working arrangement was forged between HoM and Keighley Worksafe, a trade union funded organisation that campaigned and provided information on health and safety in the workplace, and with the local Asian community centre where health checks for older Asian men became a regular occurrence, helped along by the provision of a number of delicious curries for lunch.

In July 1998 the *National Lottery Reform Bill* was passed which established a new good cause for health by providing £300 million to build a network of 'healthy living' centres in the UK. These would 'promote health and help people of all ages to maximise their well being' (National Lottery Act, 1998). In January 1999 a new distributor, the New Opportunities Fund (NOF), was formally launched to allocate funds for this purpose. From January 1999 it invited bids for the healthy living centres and enabled distributors to solicit applications from where they were not spontaneously forthcoming.

Bradford held the first meeting of the group that was to promote healthy living networks in the city in March 1999, at which we were confronted by what seemed to be the forbidding 'North face' of bureaucracy and a process that would occupy us for the next few years. Our guide up this savage route was a man whose previous incarnation as a mental health professional gave his current avatar as healthy living centre coordinator the professional skills to persistently rescue our mental health during the journey.

We completed the first stage application by October 1999 and then employed an accountant to give our philosophical musings financial credibility. The bulk of the application was so short of hard evidence that it was based mostly upon assumptions. For example, from the original project programme of activities: 'We have assumed that men will access services which are provided in a convenient place at an appropriate time.'

By August 2001 we had a business plan for *A Comprehensive Men's Health Service for the Metropolitan District of Bradford*, which we presented to the Lottery. Our numbers came up in 2002. The grant offer was accepted on the 18th April by the then Chief Executive of Bradford Metropolitan District Countil. The application to NOF was approved on the 25th April and we were in the money to the tune of just under a million pounds!

In structural terms, HoM anticipated the return to a local authority coterminous with NHS primary care and partnership working. HoM also appeared to anticipate a more holistic approach rather than a condition or illness approach to health.

Sudden wealth can be as much a curse as a blessing. Current research into wellbeing and happiness is beginning to show that since the 1970s, although gross national product has risen steadily, contentment levels have remained the same – we are richer but no happier. Lottery winners, despite an initial flood of euphoria, tend to return to previous levels of contentment when they become habituated to their wealth.

Because we were now officially a Healthy Living Centre, the need to create a HoM team certainly provoked levels of unease that perhaps were always there but now came to the fore. HoM may have been a district-wide service but the majority of the HoM team worked for individual Primary Care Trusts. PCTs were at this stage barely out of nappies and just entering adolescence in developmental terms. Their managements were often to be seen stalking their boundaries, checking that work done by their staff was performed within their territories and not in those of their rivals. This propensity reared its head over and over again throughout the project, causing sometimes the suspension and sometimes the cancellation of services that HoM team members had set up in good faith in collaboration with others of the team from different PCTs.

There then came a strange lull in activity, almost as though we needed to recover from the effort involved in winning the bid, so it was not until a year later in 2003 that HoM appointed its first business coordinator. The coordinator turned out to be very good at raising the profile of HoM and entered the project for the Health and Social Care Awards in the spring of 2004; we subsequently won the 'Reducing inequalities' category, going forward to the final in London in June. Although we didn't win in London, the regional award was a massive confidence boost for the project, gaining us national recognition and giving the group a greater sense of shared identity. In a House of Commons debate on 'Men and cancer', Dr. Howard Stoate (MP for Dartford) mentioned the HoM project in respect of having won the award and as an example of good practice.

Further honour was brought to the project by a team member who won the Queen's Nursing Institute Award for his work on weight management with men from Bradford's cleansing department in 2005.

The project has expanded into many areas of work from saunas to schools, clinics to domino clubs to barber's shops, using any and all methods to engage men in their own health. Sport has proved popular, as has providing food and going into workplaces; but also some initiatives have worked despite the prevailing wisdom, finding success in health centres and other traditional healthcare settings. What the project has illustrated is that men do and will care about their health if they are approached in the right way and offered the right sort of deal.

CHAPTER 14

How to be a men's health worker

DAVID CONRAD

INTRODUCTION

A key problem in diffusing the lessons of innovative ways of delivering health care is knowing what can be generalised and what conditions are special to the pathfinder project. One essential element is the characteristics of the workers who delivered the project. Individual qualities like enthusiasm, commitment and initiative cannot be put into a service delivery plan or simply be taken for granted. They have implications for replicating the project, including recruitment, the managerial style to be adopted, and educational and development needs of staff. Reports on innovative and successful projects, however, rarely contain useful information about the qualities of the staff and their role in achieving outcomes.

During our study of men's usage of the Bradford HoM services it became apparent that it was not simply what the individual members of the team did that was important, but also how they did it. Drawing on these findings, this chapter discusses the role of health workers' skills and attributes in marketing services to men, delivering services which meet men's needs and achieving successful outcomes.

MARKETING HEALTH SERVICES TO MEN

As men are generally reluctant to seek help with their health, and young men especially are known to approach health services with some reluctance (Lloyd 2002), relying on a traditional approach to attract men is a high-risk strategy. The willingness and ability to be innovative in marketing a men's health service can therefore have a decisive impact on whether or not it becomes successfully established. When HoM workers first advertised a men's health clinic based at a health centre, for example, only one man booked in. The apparent lack of interest in the service led to mounting pressure from health professionals at the centre to close the initiative down. Rather than assuming that the poor response necessarily reflected a lack of demand, the workers rethought their marketing strategy, changing the posters to display a large glass of beer with 'Free' on the top and 'health checks for men' in smaller print underneath. The response to the service changed very quickly, with around fourteen men being seen by two practitioners in the two and a half hour sessions. What was originally a fortnightly service then had to be delivered weekly to cope with the increased demand.

Without this kind of persistence, an attribute which proved essential in many aspects of their work, the HoM team would have failed to establish many services which ultimately proved to be highly successful. There is always, however, a difficult balance to be struck between refusing to give in to a lack of immediate success and acknowledging when a particular approach is fundamentally flawed.

The example of the beer poster highlights some of the key factors involved in marketing health services to men (Pearson 2003). As well as being eye-catching and interesting, the text should be short and to the point, without an overload of information. The use of humour in disguising the true message with what at first appeared to be an advert for free beer served to make the service appear more friendly (and male friendly) than traditional health services. Displaying a poster which initially appeared to be about beer also addressed the problem of men not wishing to be seen reading health posters for fear of being negatively judged on the basis that this constituted a deviation from the dominant norms of masculine behaviour.

Whilst free beer itself was not required to increase user numbers in this case, the use of incentives for attendance can be a valuable tool in increasing services' appeal and has been employed successfully in other health projects aimed at young men (Lloyd 2002). Judging in which circumstances this will be helpful and appropriate is therefore an important skill. HoM workers successfully used the offer of a weekend trip as an incentive for teenage boys to attend health sessions at a youth centre. Rather than simply serving as an unrelated bribe, however, the preparations for the trip became a part of the boys' learning experience, engaging them in the planning as well as the organising of a sponsored walk to raise the required funds.

In order to gain access to a particular group or setting it is sometimes also necessary to market the idea of a service to gatekeepers before it can be established. A willingness to engage in this process is particularly important when setting up new services in non-traditional settings, such as places of worship. Again, persistence and tenacity are required here, as there can often be long periods before workers are invited into a particular setting.

DELIVERING SERVICES WHICH MEET MEN'S NEEDS

Although the marketing skills and an ability to take a flexible and innovative approach to publicity are very important, the uptake of any service is dependent on whether it is perceived to meet a need of its target users. Service provision must be tailored to specific groups of men. This was highlighted for the HoM team by the poor response to a drop-in event which they held at a local university. Although the service was based on a format which had already proved successful at a college and elsewhere, the offer of free condoms as an incentive proved to have much less effect on university students.

Whilst men are generally reluctant to visit health professionals, the overall success of the HoM project shows that men are concerned about their health and willing to engage with health topics in situations where they feel comfortable. The success of men's health nights and sessions in Australia (Verrinder & Denner 2000), and projects based in male friendly settings, such as football grounds (Pringle & Sayers 2004) also supports the idea that men will respond enthusiastically to services which they feel are for them. Partly this is about tackling the sense of guilt which men have over visiting the doctor for anything other than an obvious physical problem (Richardson & Rabiee 2001):

> . . . you know guys will come in to see you and the classic stuff. They don't want to waste the GP's time; they feel as though if they go and see the doctor when they're feeling well they'd be a complete fraud really. But once they've seen you, and whether their BP's high, or whether they're obese or whether they're putting weight on, whatever, they feel quite justified in going to see the doctor or the practice nurse or whoever. But you know, in either case people will pass the GP to come and see you at a drop-in somewhere, and then happily go and see the GP. (HoM Key Worker)

Being seen to be non-judgemental is important both for engaging service users and encouraging initial attendance. Users of the HoM services expressed concerns about negative reactions which they might receive from health professionals who might consider their concerns to be trivial:

> . . . they find it hard to go to say 'Well, I'm feeling fine but could you just check my blood pressure?' or 'I'd like my cholesterol checking.' And then sometimes maybe the response they've had in the past from, whether it be a nurse or a doctor, as in 'Well, you're OK, you don't need it doing.' . . . They never seem to be encouraged to take a proactive stance in their health, whether that's unintentional from the non-verbal signs they pick up from the nurse or the doctor that they go and see. (HoM Key Worker)

Whilst men have a tendency to talk about specific problems when visiting health professionals (Tudiver & Talbot 1999), HoM workers employed a holistic, rather than medical, approach to health. Placing the emphasis on solutions instead of focussing on health problems has also been found to be a more effective way of engaging men (Lloyd 2002). This shifts the message from being a negative one ('you use this service because you have a problem') to something more positive and optimistic ('using this service will help you to avoid problems and improve your quality of life'). Framing the delivery of health services in a positive way is particularly important when working with men because it tackles the feeling that in utilising them they would effectively be labelling themselves as ill. The perception of health services as 'illness services' discourages men from attending those which are aimed at preventing ill health by achieving behaviour change; it also creates an association between the usage of health services and the acknowledgement of illness, which men tend to perceive as an act of weakness.

Health care has traditionally been delivered in health clinics where professionals have configured services for their own convenience. The expectation is that the patient will learn to use the service and will conform to its structures and ways of working. Bringing health services to men requires a reversal of this expectation – going into the men's own environment and engaging with them on their terms. One of the most important attributes of the HoM team was their willingness to take health services to the men, rather than setting up services and simply waiting for men to come to them. This is because men are not only reluctant to access health services directly, but also tend to be restricted by their work requirements.

With health centres closing early and not opening at weekends, there are increasing barriers to working men's ability to access clinics. This is a particular problem for men as they are more likely to be working full time, more likely to be working more than 48 hours a week and are less likely to have a job that involves flexitime (DoH 2004a). Users of the HoM services frequently referred to the need to make appointments in order to see a GP and felt that health centres were not accessible for men, either in terms of location or opening hours:

> You say to your employer that you want some time off to go to the doctor's, the first thing they will say is, 'why, what's up?' And often this is in an open area, not all bosses would take you into an office, shut the door and have a one-to-one chat, it depends on your relationship with your managers but for many men the boss is still the boss and he has a lot of control over what happens in your life. So any signs of weakness . . . say there is redundancy and I have been to the doctor three times in the last couple of months, are they going to find a way of getting me out, am I at risk of getting sick? It reflects on men's ability and their vision of themselves. (HoM Key Worker)

Linked with this is another significant barrier to men's utilisation of health services – the issue of control. Traditional notions of masculinity place a high value on the maintenance of control, independence and freedom. Addis and Mahalik (2003) point out that the loss of control involved in visiting a doctor can be multifaceted, including being made to wait to be seen, having to follow instructions for treatment and having the body subjected to medical examinations and procedures. These indignities are endured for the privilege of being told, in most cases by someone of greater social status who knows more about the patient's body than they do, that their body is out of their control and rendering a failure their attempts to live up to their own idea of masculine identity. From this perspective, it is not difficult to rationalise men's general reluctant to visit their GPs.

Delivering services which minimise this loss of control for users whilst still achieving valid outcomes requires a flexible approach from men's health workers. As well as taking services into environments where men feel comfortable, offering drop-in rather than appointment-based services wherever appropriate can reduce the need for service users to hand over control. Examples from the HoM work include the *Lads' Room*, an information shop for young lads in which a HoM worker would be available to provide contraceptives and health advice two days a week, and the barber shop health MOTs which allowed men to have a health check whilst waiting for a haircut.

Successfully devising, setting up and marketing new men's health services clearly requires certain skills in addition to those which are needed simply to run existing programmes. Instead of simply delivering health services in accordance with established protocols, the HoM team have adopted the role of entrepreneurs – creating something new and different which changes values (Faugier 2005).

ACHIEVING OUTCOMES

Setting up services which men will access does not of course constitute an end in itself. The success of a project depends on how well it engages users in order to meet its stated objectives. One of the ways that this can be achieved is by giving the men an opportunity to reciprocate by helping each other in a group situation, rather than simply being the recipients of help (Addis & Mahalik 2003). This serves to counter the perception that the user's role is based on a passive state of weakness that contradicts the traditional masculine identity of strength and independence.

Framing tasks as competition is a good way of enabling reciprocity among users and creating a sense of shared experience which utilises the traditional male gender identity. The HoM team used this strategy very effectively with their weight loss programmes, with participants being split into teams and competing to lose weight.

The extent to which men will engage with health sessions depends largely on how well they are able to engage with the workers who are running them. A strength of the HoM team was their ability to gain the confidence of the men and to be accepted as individuals that could be trusted. Adopting a non-threatening style, smiling and using appropriate humour to break the ice, whilst maintaining a professional affect, are key: *'This chap said to me, "I think if someone told me that if I don't stop [smoking] I will die, then I would stop." so I said, "Okay, if you don't stop you will die!".'* (HoM Key Worker)

The willingness and ability to empathise with men is essential for engaging them with health messages in a sustained and meaningful way. In part, this is achieved by not being tied to a medical model of seeing the service users as patients with problems: *'When I have done group work with men it comes across to me that we are ordinary blokes, and ordinary blokes are what ordinary blokes relate to . . .'* (HoM Key Worker)

HoM workers acknowledged that whilst engaging men often required them to behave, as one user put it, *'like a mate'* there was a constant need to balance this with the need to maintain the role of the professional. One of the workers recounted working with young lads early in his career:

> . . . *when I was in the group I would try too much to be part of it by swearing and being more profane than the rest of them, 'cause I had just started doing this work and tried to be part of the gang. And the youth worker who had more experience afterwards said, 'What are you doing . . . ? You're not one of the lads, you know.' And I realised that's what I was trying to do – I was trying to be one of the lads and I couldn't be because I wasn't.* (HoM Key Worker)

Maintaining a positive attitude towards service users is essential. Working effectively with men requires a willingness to take time to engage with them and accept that for many the threat to their masculine identity of acknowledging problems is a genuine barrier which will not be overcome during a single consultation. A tactic which has been found to be successful in enabling young men to address health problems without feeling 'less of a man' is to offer sociological explanations for them, shifting the emphasis away from the concept of something being 'wrong' with the individual (Lloyd 2002).

In dealing with men in a way which is sympathetic to traditional aspects of masculine identity, so as to engage them and help to make them comfortable in dealing with health issues, there is of course a danger of legitimising and reinforcing the traditional notions of masculinity which have been a negative influence on men's attitudes to health. Finding a balance between the two will never be easy, however anyone aiming to change men's attitudes towards masculinity as a prerequisite for increasing their usage of services will inevitably find themselves blowing against a very strong wind.

Keeping a realistic sense of what can be achieved is important through all stages of setting up and delivering a men's health service. For one member of the HoM team, a reduction in the number of times he was told to 'f***' off was an indication of success.

MOVING FORWARD

Many of the skills which workers need to successfully deliver men's health services, such as adopting a non-threatening approach and balancing the role of the professional with a use of 'blokey' language and humour, can be taught or learnt through practical experience. Also, there seems to be no evidence that workers necessarily need to be male. Users of the HoM services tended to express remarkably little interest in the question of female workers delivering men's health sessions: *'It wouldn't bother me at all, no. It could be a bloody alien for me. You know, I'm not bothered as long as it's going to help me. That's the main point, isn't it?'* (HoM Service User, aged 33).

Whilst there is currently a shortage of people who possess the necessary skills to deliver services on the ground, this is not because competent men's health workers constitute a 'special breed' whose numbers are kept low by the rare nature of their personal qualities. Once protocols for men's health services are established, there are no fundamentally insurmountable barriers to successfully recruiting workers to deliver them.

The work of the HoM team shows that establishing workable protocols for successful men's health services does, however, require individuals who possess entrepreneurial skills which are out of the ordinary. It would clearly be impractical and unrealistic to base the rolling out of a men's health programme on a plan of exclusively recruiting workers in possession of these additional skills to run the services. The future therefore lies in utilising the skills and experiences of entrepreneurial men's health workers, such as the Bradford HoM team, to develop standardised models for men's health services which can then be rolled out on a national basis.

CONCLUSION

The success of the HoM project has largely been due to the qualities and attributes of the key workers who have set up and delivered the services. Persistence (the ability to stick to an approach); flexibility (the ability to drop an approach when it is not working); and being non-judgemental (neutrality in the face of the service users' actions and beliefs) have proved to be particularly important in engaging men and boys.

Whilst only a small proportion of health workers will possess the entrepreneurial skills required to conceive of and establish new types of men's health services, the skills required to deliver those services in accordance with existing protocols can be taught or learned fairly straightforwardly through practice. There are, however, important implications for the way that pioneering projects are run: managers must be comfortable with flexibility and some uncertainty and there has to be an openness of teamwork to enable useful evaluations of progress to be made. In all men's health projects, staff development and education should be focussed on building the relevant skills and qualities required for successfully and efficiently engaging with boys and men.

CHAPTER 15

'It'll be alright on the night' – the everyday pitfalls of delivering men's health services

NICK DAVY, CHRIS BRADLEY, ANDREW HARRISON AND PETE WESTWOOD

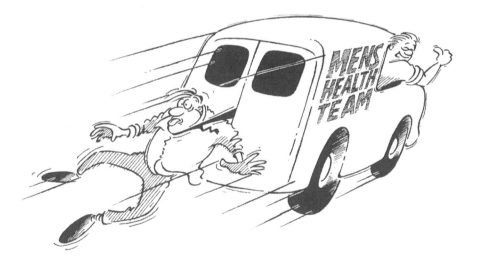

INTRODUCTION

Following the tips in this book should dramatically increase your chances of success in setting up health services for men and boys, but it would be wrong to give the impression that there's a set of rules which will guarantee plain sailing. A key factor in the success of the HoM project has been the workers' ability to take hiccups and disasters in their stride, remain determined, know when to give up (and when not to give up) and to continually learn from both the triumphs and the disasters.

To prepare the reader for some of the everyday challenges which they might face, this chapter provides a few personal reflections from some of the HoM workers on things which haven't completely gone according to plan.

NICK DAVY

A few years ago, we started drop-ins at the same time at both a local college and a university. The two sites are only a few hundred metres apart and were both similarly promoted, actually more promoted at the university as we were at the Freshers' Fair handing out free condoms and telling people about the new service. Just about from day one the drop-in at the college was accessed and within three months we were averaging ten contacts for a two hour drop-in. After the same time we had only had one person accessing the drop-in at the university during each two hour period. We had what we thought was a favourable location at the university, i.e. above the bar, and continued to place small cards promoting the drop-in around the university, including in the bar.

One vitally important thing to know with regard to the development of drop-ins is to give them time to build, as was demonstrated by the drop-in at the information shop for young people mentioned elsewhere in this book. After a year we were averaging about two people accessing this service weekly but after five years we now average fifteen for the same time period. This demonstrates that word of mouth is vital to the development of such services.

By the end of the first year the college drop-in continued to grow in popularity and the total number of people accessing the university drop-in had risen to two! Obviously there comes a point where one has to assess the effectiveness of time and resources and after discussion with partners involved we decided to stop the university drop-in to concentrate on more productive areas of work.

We have thought long and hard about the contrast between the two drop-ins; maybe university students are financially better off and therefore the draw of free condoms isn't so effective, maybe university students are more confident about accessing services through GPs and have greater knowledge of local services or maybe university students are less concerned about pregnancy and STIs or maybe don't have sex! We obviously don't know why there was such a difference in the uptake of the same service in similar environments and would welcome any theories!

One large area of work which can vary enormously as regards success is puberty and sex and relationship work in schools. We have sometimes been asked to deliver sessions in primary and upper schools where the teachers quite clearly see it as an opportunity to catch up on some marking at the back of the class or simply to have a break and recharge their batteries! I remember one set of horror sessions where we were asked to deliver five sessions to upper school lads simply, I feel sure, so the school could 'tick the box' and say it had been done. The teacher sat at the back of a class of 25–30 lads saying nothing and not getting involved at all, and every ten minutes or so as the behaviour became more uncontrollable he would shout at the top of his voice, totally unconstructively, send a lad out who happened to be the last one to act up, sit down, continue to do nothing for another ten minutes and then repeat his previous behaviour! I would be very reluctant to work with this size group now with increased knowledge of how lads can behave in larger groups. I would always try to negotiate to have more time in the school and have smaller, more productive groups.

This demonstrates to me how important it is to plan sessions with the teacher who will be supporting me in the class. The teacher has the advantage of knowing the lads individually and is also far more skilled than me in controlling a class. The vast majority of teachers we work with are committed to delivering this work in as productive manner as possible but pre-planning is vital to the success of such sessions.

CHRIS BRADLEY

When I started working in schools I had long hair and a pony tail. In two or three different schools I was called "miss" by the young children for the whole session, despite my protests. In challenging stereotypes we always told the kids we were nurses and this often met with laughter because they almost all believed that nurses were all women and men became doctors.

In a pub in Keighley in the early days we ran a pub quiz with a £20 prize after a single dads' football tournament. A young man sitting on his own won with every question correctly answered and I went over and gave him the prize, also asking for feedback on what he thought of the quiz. His response was direct to the point of aggression: 'It was s***, now f*** off.' Another lesson – men respond in an almost infinite variety of ways to the health message.

I recall telling a health visitor more or less the same thing when I was a lorry driver many years ago, because I felt she was the voice of the establishment spying on my family, despite the fact that she had never visited us before. I lived in Selby at the time so if she is reading this (though she will be retired by now I would think) and recalls an unnecessarily aggressive man on Westbourne Road throwing her out, this is my apology. I was just being a man in the only way I knew.

I recall when we used to visit schools and talk to primary age children about the emotional and physical changes of growing up they quickly adapted from the tradition of only girls having this talk to boys having one as well. It was apparently traditionally called the 'Tampax lesson' and I wondered what they now secretly called it. I found out when out shopping, when I was introduced to a mum as 'This is the man who comes to school and does sex with us'. A quiet word with this mum soon sorted it out, but it could have got uncomfortable.

On another occasion, my colleague and I were out in the main street of our small town when we were spotted by a group of teenage boys who we had been talking to about testicular cancer self checking. As a greeting they shouted across the road our slogan 'Know your balls, check 'em out', adopted from the educational video we used.

Possibly our most memorable failure was one of our early drop-ins. We had done the market research and found a very accessible place in a local recreation centre. We even contributed from our funds to improving the premises and put up signs all over the place advertising when and where to find us. Response was poor, with most clients being repeat visitors. We laid on refreshments, readvertised, altered the signs, changed the times to evenings and nothing happened. The idea never took off on that site despite being successful at other places. The problem was probably to do with traditional associations with the site and the park outside. Gangs of youths gather there and street crime is associated with the area. Location, location, location!

Schools work is fraught with danger, even with younger children. Survival tips from my experience include:

- Keep groups to a manageable size, however much schools plead for bigger groups.
- Don't try to be 'one of the lads', it doesn't work and it doesn't impress. It also gives pupils permission to act any way they choose.
- Always have a member of school staff in the room, preferably one the lads are fairly relaxed with. I once worked with a games master present, as the session was held during his lesson. It was bad enough that the lads would rather have been playing football, but within a few minutes this teacher had *me* scared of him – not much chance of getting questions about what their main concerns were, then?
- Don't do favours. We once travelled 80 miles in our own time to demonstrate our outreach work in school for a schoolteacher friend. This had to be done voluntarily because it was so far out of our area, but it was a personal favour. The group we talked to was huge, crammed into too small a room. There was no opportunity for interaction and insufficient time for questions so we invited written questions and answered them all later. We persuaded someone from another organisation to join us, making the team three strong. We travelled for over three hours, prepared for four hours and delivered for over an hour. We replied to all the questions in our spare time. We charged £60.00 for the session, which almost covered travel costs. Not surprisingly, we had a request for the same session the following year. I calculated the true cost to be around £750 and declined the booking.
- As in all presentations, preparation is almost everything. I once delivered a talk to a group of GPs in their study protected learning time. I returned from annual leave to be handed the task – 'Don't worry, you'll easily do it from your head, it's just about access to services'. I should have continued to resist – it was the worst session I have ever attended, let alone delivered. I was embarrassed and unprepared and the GPs were not impressed at giving up their time to listen to this nonsense. And we billed them for the time.

❭ Don't be afraid to talk to adults as adults. The best session we ever delivered to staff groups about our work was based on role-plays of teenagers using street language. It was repeated on request on several occasions far and wide. The only safe ship is one that doesn't leave the harbour.

ANDREW HARRISON

Following work in various youth centres and schools, lads had been encouraged to call at the clinic if they wanted condoms. Generally, if my window was open it was a sign that I was in, the lads would call up and I'd go downstairs to meet them. On one occasion I could hear this boy shouting 'Andrew' and he seemed very near. When I turned to go to the window to say I'd be coming down, there he was. He had shinned up the drainpipe and his face was squashed against the window as he clung on for dear life.

Distributing condoms from outside the clinic door received horrified looks from the lead nurse, who was concerned about the local paper sensationalising it. The lead nurse had arrived for a meeting at the same time as a group of lads had turned up on their bikes requesting condoms. I was told at a later date about these concerns and asked if we could get the lads to come in, sit round a desk and work 'more formally'.

When I first started to work with the team I was asked to support a community health day to promote men's health drop-ins. Up until this point these particular services were not well utilised. Two colleagues (one of whom has since moved on) came to lend a hand. One spent quite a while chatting to a group of lads who had just finished playing football. He was quite excited and reckoned that his 'chat' would encourage the lads to use the service at the youth centre. However, when he turned around it was evident that the lads were less impressed as they had stuck a sign on his back . . . 'F*** off you t***'. Everyone cracked up, and it did begin a working relationship with this particular group.

We did a chaotic first aid session with a group of young men at a youth centre. The group found it hard to concentrate on their work as some of their mates were outside hanging from the windows like chimps, shouting abuse and giving everyone the 'V' sign. When the group was asked 'What would you do if you found someone collapsed?' the group response was 'Pinch his wallet and get his mobile'.

We organised a partnership event for dads and their children with a health visitor. Quite a bit of planning had gone into the event and it was envisaged (going from the return slips) that plenty of men would turn up. The 51-seater coach turned up to take the group away, but not one of the dads appeared.

Food diaries – a guy had been religiously completing his food diary for the practice nurse and couldn't understand why he wasn't losing weight. The diary read: 'Weetabix for breakfast, ham sandwich for lunch and tuna pasta for evening meal'. I visited the guy, just as he was preparing his tuna pasta . . . which was being mixed in a huge washing up bowl! Portion sizes needed to be discussed.

The *Retired Men's Forum* – quite a lot of work went into a joint session with the *Walking for Health* coordinator. This group of approximately 30 men had requested our input and so we delivered and promoted health issues with the aim of creating a healthy eating and exercise class. At the end only one person expressed an interest – the treasurer's wife. The men reckoned they didn't have long to live and any changes in lifestyle weren't really worth the effort.

PETE WESTWOOD

Setting up *Weight Management* and *Stop Smoking* groups at a chemical company – despite a lengthy face to face meeting with the company contact, numerous emails and a programme of MoTs delivered by the HoM team to almost 100 of the male employees, our *Weight Management* group for men on the first week consisted of seven women and two men! The clue was that the team's name was Health of **Men**! When we pointed out to our contact who had recruited the clients that this wasn't what we had expected/envisioned, she still couldn't see what was wrong! I suppose the moral of the story is that while the contact/link person in the workplace *is* indeed an invaluable resource, we do need to be crystal clear about our expectations and not assume that our understanding of men's health issues is replicated in other health professionals' mindsets!

When ground rules have been agreed with teenagers on a weekend residential regarding a ban on drinking alcohol, avoid indulging yourself, or, failing that, make sure that you don't get caught!

Never, **ever** deliver a puberty session to 60 boys all at once! Just say no!

Make sure that whatever innovations occur or whatever good work is done, that it is written up and preferably published – before someone else does!

CHAPTER 16

Conclusion

ALAN WHITE AND DAVID CONRAD

INTRODUCTION

The challenges men face with their health are clear, with the data showing men are at a significantly higher risk of dying prematurely from a wide range of health issues. Though it is apparent that the overall life expectancy for men is increasing, this seems to be predominately in the professional classes, but even there they have only just reached the level that women in the same social class were at 30 years ago and so complacency should be strenuously avoided. For the manual blue collar worker and those men who have not been able to enter the labour market or have been made redundant the situation is far from satisfactory, with increased levels of morbidity and mortality leading to some areas of the country with life expectancies amongst the lowest in Europe.

We know that in society there is a large proportion of men who have disease that has not been identified. The number of men with undiagnosed hypertension is estimated at 22.6%, and 1% of the population has undiagnosed diabetes. The problem of the overweight male, with its increased risks due to metabolic syndrome, is also overlooked by many practitioners, with a failure to address it seriously.

The problems that many men face with their health goes beyond these disease states, with difficulties experienced in relation to their roles as fathers and as supporters of partners with long-term conditions. It is a complex world that we live in now and it seems that the socialisation process men and boys are subjected to gives little protection when things begin to go wrong.

The data shows that men are particularly vulnerable in times of transition, especially if this results in some form of loss, for instance divorce, separation from their children, redundancy, retirement, death of a spouse, even the increasing incidence of speeding fines (leading to a large proportion of men that do not see themselves as bad drivers being at risk of losing their driving licences). Managing such stress often results in emotional problems that materialise through alcohol or drug misuse, smoking, reduced efficiency, lowered self-esteem, irritability and even violence and suicide (Brownhill *et al.* 2005).

FINDING A SOLUTION

Though work in this growing field of men's health is still in its infancy we are able to suggest that part of the problem is due to the way men access and use the NHS (White 2001; Robertson 2003; O'Brien *et al.*, 2005). Or, put another way, the NHS as it is currently configured seems to be alienating to a significant proportion of the population!

Whilst we appreciate the argument that there has been in place, since the inception of the NHS in the 1940s, a service that is open to all, the data seems to suggest that this may not be as universal as first thought. With almost twice as many men as women working full time, with many having little access to flexitime and now a high proportion working over 48 hours a week, often away from home, getting to a nine-to-five service is nigh on impossible. If it is difficult to access when sick then the chances of accessing it for a health check is even more of a challenge. This would not be a problem if it were not for the disproportionately high levels of premature death as a result of what should be, in the current era, preventable causes.

Men are becoming increasingly aware of their health needs such that although up to now there has been little pressure for services to be male friendly there is the possibility that this will increase in the future. There is in addition the added impetus for change now that the new gender duty is in force. With its requirement to meet the different needs of men and women there is a legally binding impetus for action on these currently problematic services. If these services were extended into the evening and open at weekends many more men (and women) could access them, but the interviews with the men using the HoM services have suggested that this is not enough. There also needs to be consideration given to the appointments system and the way men (particularly young men and men in distress) are made welcome in an arena that is currently seen as predominately focussed on women, young children and the elderly. We must recognise though that many men would still be reluctant users of the NHS as a consequence of a socialisation process that models itself on independence and avoiding admitting to vulnerabilities. With these arguably being therefore the most at risk of harbouring hidden health problems, alternative methods of targeting them must be considered. It is within this area that the work outlined within this book becomes not just a model for Bradford but for male focussed provision elsewhere as well.

What the team in Bradford has done is to show that it is possible to creatively work outside of the conventional health care services to target men where they are. The examples in this book give those who are looking for ways to engage with men ideas that have been grounded in practice. What the team have created is a wealth of experience in going out into communities and setting up services that work.

The ideas outlined in this book will also provide guidance for those who are developing plans for meeting the need to promote self-care within the general population. Being able to reach men has a huge pay-off with regard to improving the health of the nation. For not only does it create healthier males, through increasing men's awareness of health it will also enable them to be more engaged with their families' health needs.

OTHER WORK IN THE AREA

The Bradford team have been in an excellent position to develop new services as a result of the Big Lottery funding, however there are many other examples of innovative services being developed around the UK. The largest development has been in Scotland where the work of Leishman and Dalziel, who developed the Camelon Centre for Men's Health, was used as a model to develop a series of pilot sites across the country with a £4m government grant. The Camelon service provided appointment based individual physical and emotional health assessments which include BP, urine and cholesterol checks, and information on the prostate gland and testicular examination. The service also provided weight and stress management groups, health information and education.

Another substantial initiative was undertaken in Preston with a Men's Health Initiative. The project was managed by community nurses and health promotion specialists but had a different focus from the Bradford team's, supporting a wide range of community based projects, which included:

» *Owd Lads and Young Lads* project
» Nurse led research clinics
» Asian men's homeless worker
» African-Caribbean men's worker
» Young gay and bisexual men's project.

This initiative was evaluated by a research team from Liverpool John Moores University who identified that the most successful projects incorporated:

» Accessibility and coverage
» Sustainable activities
» Practical, long-term outcomes
» Quality of life through sustainable support networks
» Provision of access to other services
» Integrated projects and partnership working
» Reflexive and reflective working practices
» Good communication
» Transferable skills and practices
» Outreach.

(Kierans 2006)

Away from these large projects the majority of work has been undertaken by individuals who have been able to develop novel approaches, with DeVille-Almond seen by many as one of the key pioneers of alternative provision for men. She set up the first barber shop service and has expanded her work to include the setting up of health clinics within settings where men are likely to congregate including:

> Pub clinics
> Harley-Davidson showroom *Bikers and Health*
> *Goodwood Festival of Speed* men's health clinic
> *GI's* barber shop men's health clinic
> *Lymm Truck Stop* surgery.

(DeVille-Almond 2007)

Now working as an independent nurse consultant, DeVille-Almond has mainly focussed on men and their weight, but through this approach has been able to identify many men with previously undiagnosed health problems.

Working with a specific group of men known to have a health risk was a central part of the success of McCullagh's *Tommy the Trucker* project in Sefton. There the focus was on a healthy living campaign for lorry drivers who work at the Port of Liverpool, whose long hours in a cab lead to an increased risk of obesity amongst other emotional and physical difficulties.

Other approaches that have been developed include the work of Hopkins (2001), who recognised the limited resources for young lads and developed resources that could be used to get across messages relating to safe sex, puberty and mental health problems. Some of these were in the form of comics, for instance *Boyz Will be Boyz* and *Men-tal*; others have been developed outside of the NHS to allow for more freedom in using language and imagery that the lads will understand, but would be too challenging for mainstream health services (in much the same way that the Terrence Higgins Trust was able to speak the language of the gay community in getting across health messages about HIV/AIDS in the 1980s). The *Red Knob* work can be found at www.theredknob.com.

Using imagery to target men specifically has also been adopted by O'Brien, who uses the concept of social marketing to devise health campaigns. Based in Knowsley, his work includes the *Pit Stop* for men aged 50–65 years to have a health check, which was advertised using car imagery.

Further good use of male-specific spaces has been made by practitioners who have teamed up with football and rugby clubs. The Football Association is very keen to see their resources used for the benefit of communities and now have specific ambassadors for health, including Tony Adams, a footballer who himself had mental health problems, now being their campaigner for mental health.

One successful project is found at Manchester United football ground where men with emotional problems are supported to use an environment where they feel at home and safe and can explore their own difficulties using terms associated with football to understand their problems and to find solutions (www.itsagoal.org.uk). The originator of the programme, a Cheshire-based social entrepreneur, developed the project at Macclesfield football ground before it was taken up at the Old Trafford site, with a community psychiatric nurse working with the men on managing the programme (Pringle & Sayers 2004).

Targeting men through the web has also been used successfully. Recognising that many men find it difficult to access health care, either through their work patterns or through a reluctance to seek help, the web has been found to be a key source of easily accessed information for men, with the added benefit of being anonymous (Pollard 2007). Charities such as the Prostate Cancer Charity, the Orchid Foundation and the British Heart Foundation have all provided extremely important sources of information for men on their disease states, with studies that have been conducted with men showing how many gather significant amounts of information about their condition and treatment options (Kelsey *et al.* 2004).

The Bradford HoM team have their own successful website (www.healthofmen. org) that attracted over 300,000 hits in 2004 and covers a broader range of health issues than the disease-specific sites. Another key site for the man on the street to gain impartial advice on their health is found at the Men's Health Forum website (www.malehealth.co.uk). This site has received a number of awards and commendations for its clarity and breadth of authoritative coverage, including the Royal Society of Medicine Medical Website of the Year 2004.

The Men's Health Forum has also been involved in the development of a number of books aimed at men using the format of car repair manuals in conjunction with publishers Haynes (Banks 2002; Banks 2004; Banks 2004a; Banks 2005; Banks 2006). Four of the series have been directly linked to the theme of the yearly *Men's Health Week* that runs up to Father's Day in June. These have also been award winners, both in terms of plain English and in terms of clarity of their health messages for men.

TAKING THE PLUNGE

For anyone wishing to set up community based services for men, the initiatives described in Part Two provide great examples of what can be achieved, but you shouldn't be afraid to create your own projects based on the same basic principles. Whenever it's appropriate, you should look for ways to go to the men and deliver services on *their* terms rather than waiting for them to come and find you, but don't expect men to want to talk about their continence problems while they're having a pint or waiting for a haircut! Not all your ducklings will turn into swans, but don't give up if you don't see immediate results.

The key messages to take away from this book are: be innovative, be flexible, be determined and you *can* deliver health services which men *will* want to use. The lessons in this book don't represent a set of 'golden rules' which will guarantee success every time, but they will help to dramatically improve your strike rate. Good luck!

References

Addis M and Mahalik JR (2003) Men, masculinity, and the contexts of help seeking. *Am Psychol*. **58**: 5–14

Arber S, Price D, Davidson K and Perren K (2003) Re-examining gender and marital status: material well-being and social involvement. In: Arber S, Davidson K and Ginn J (eds) *Gender and Ageing: changing roles and relationships*. Maidenhead: Open University Press.

ASH (2006) http://www.ash.org.uk/html/factsheets/html/basic01.html [Accessed 29/1/07].

Banks I (2002) *The Man Manual*. Sparkford: JH Haynes & Co. Ltd.

Banks I (2004) *Cancer: any age, any time*. Sparkford: JH Haynes & Co. Ltd.

Banks I (2004a) *The Women Manual: the practical step-by-step guide to women's health, for men*. Sparkford: JH Haynes & Co. Ltd.

Banks I (2005) *HGV Man Manual: reducing all large sizes, all shapes and colours*. Sparkford: JH Haynes & Co. Ltd.

Banks I (2006) *Brain Manual: the step-by-step guide for men to achieving and maintaining mental well-being*. Sparkford: JH Haynes & Co. Ltd.

Bradbeer C, Soni S, Ekbote A and Martin T (2006) You're not going to give me the umbrella, are you? *BMJ*. **333**: 1287–1288.

British Heart Foundation (2003) *Written evidence to the Health Select Committee*. London: British Heart Foundation.

British Medical Journal. *Best Treatments – clinical evidence for patients from the BMJ* [Internet]. Available from: http://www.besttreatments.co.uk [Accessed 12/9/06].

Brownhill S, Wilhelm K, Barclay L and Schmied V (2005) 'Big build': hidden depression in men. *Austr N Z J Psychiatry*. **39**: 921–931.

BUPA (2006) *Attention deficit hyperactivity disorder (ADHD) in children* [Internet]. Available from: http://hcd2.bupa.co.uk/fact_sheets/html/attention_deficit.html [Accessed 12/8/06].

Combined Homelessness and Information Network (CHAIN) (2005) *Rough Sleeping Report for London 2004/5*. London: CHAIN.

Commission for Racial Equality (CRE). *Race equality impact assessment – Statistics: Health care services* [Internet]. Available from: http://www.cre.gov.uk/duty/reia/statistics_health.html [Accessed 20/9/06].

Connell RW (1995) *Masculinities*. Oxford: Polity Press.

Costain L (2003) *Diet Trials: how to succeed at dieting*. London: BBC Books.

Courtenay WH (2000) Constructions of masculinity and their influence on men's well-being: a theory of gender and health. *Soc Sci Med*. **50**: 1385–1401.

Courtney WH, McCreary DR and Merighi JR (2002) Gender and ethnic differences in health beliefs and behaviours. *J Health Psychol*. **7**: 219–231.

Davidson K and Arber S (2003) Older men's health: a life course issue? *Men's Health Journal*. **2**: 72–75.

Department for Education and Employment (2000) *Sex and Relationship Education Guidance*. London: DfEE.

Department of Health (1998) *Smoking Kills*. London: DoH.

Department of Health (1999) *The Health of Minority Ethnic Groups: health survey for England*. London: DoH.

Department of Health (2001) *Better Prevention, Better Services, Better Sexual Health. The National Strategy for Sexual Health and HIV*. London: DoH. http://www.dh.gov.uk/en/Consultations/Closedconsultations/DH 4084674 [Accessed 10/10/06].

Department of Health (2003a) *Contraception and Sexual Health*. London: DoH.

Department of Health (2003b) *Effective Sexual Health Promotion*. London: DoH.

Department of Health (2003c) *Health Survey for England 2002*. London: DoH.

Department of Health (2004a) *Health Survey for England 2003*. London: DoH.

Department of Health (2004b) *Choosing Health: making healthier choices easier*. London: DoH.

Department of Health (2005) *Health Survey for England 2004: the health of minority ethnic groups – headline tables*. London: DoH.

Department of Health (2006) *Our Health, Our Care, Our Say: a new direction for community services*. London: DoH.

Department of Trade and Industry (2005) *Advancing Equality for Men and Women: Government proposals to introduce a public sector duty to promote gender equality*. London: Department of Trade and Industry.

DeVille-Almond J (2002) Innovations in men's health: working 'outside the box'. *Men's Health Journal*. **1**: 88–90.

DeVille-Almond J (2007) Innovation in obesity services for men. In: White AK and Pettifer M (eds) *Hazardous Waist: tackling male weight problems*. Oxford: Radcliffe.

DfES (2006) http://www.dfes.gov.uk/rsgateway/DB/SBU/b000209/980-t3.htm [Accessed 29/1/07].

DrugScope (2006) *New figures reveal reduction in drug-related deaths* [Internet]. Available from: http://www.drugscope.org.uk/news_item.asp?intID=1374 [Accessed 8/11/06].

Elliott J (2005) *'Accidental check-up saved my life.'* http://news.bbc.co.uk/1/hi/health/4565069.stm

Equality Act 2006. London: HMSO.

Faugier J (2005) Developing a new generation of nurse entrepreneurs. *Nurs Stand.* **19**: 49–53.

Freund P and McGuire M (1991) *Health, Illness and the Social Body.* Englewood Cliffs, NJ: Prentice Hall.

Frosh S, Phoenix A and Pattman R (2002) *Young Masculinities: understanding boys in contemporary society.* Basingstoke: Palgrave.

Galdas P, Cheater MF and Marshall P (2005) Men and health help-seeking behaviour: literature review. *J Adv Nurs.* **49**: 616–23.

Garfinkel H (1967) *Studies in Ethnomethodology.* Englewood Cliffs, NJ: Prentice Hall.

Goddard E (2005) *(General Household Survey 2005) Smoking and drinking among adults, 2005.* London: Office for National Statistics.

Gray J (1993) *Men are from Mars, Women are from Venus.* London: Thorsons.

Green J (1999) *The Big Book of Filth: 6500 sex slang words and phrases.* London: Cassell.

Health Development Agency (2002) *Boys' and Young Men's Health: what works?* London: HDA.

Health Development Agency (2003) *Teenage Parenting and Parenthood: a review of reviews.* London: HDA.

Health Protection Agency (2005) *Mapping the Issues: HIV and other Sexually Transmitted Infections in the United Kingdom: 2005.* London: HPA.

Hopkins P (2001) Boys will be men. *Nurs Times.* **97**: 26–27.

Independent Advisory Group on Sexual Health and HIV (2005) *Annual Report: 2004/2005.* London: DoH.

Jarvis MJ and Wardle J (1999) Social patterning of individual health behaviours: the case of cigarette smoking. In: Marmot MG and Wilkinson RG (eds) *Social Determinants of Health.* Oxford: Oxford University Press.

Kelsey S, Owens J and White AK (2004) The experience of radiotherapy for localised prostate cancer: the men's perspective. *Eur J Cancer Care.* **13**: 272–278.

Key TJ, Schatzkin A, Willett WC, Allen NE, Spencer EA and Travis R (2004) Diet, nutrition and the prevention of cancer. *Public Health Nutr.* **7** Supplement 1: 187–200.

Kierans C (2006) *Masculinity, Health and Use of Health Services.* Preston: European Men's Health Development Foundation.

Kirby RS and Kirby MG (2004) Benign and malignant diseases of the prostate. In: Kirby RS, Carson CC, Kirby MG and Farah RN (eds) *Men's Health.* 2nd ed. London: Martin Dunitz.

'Know Your Balls . . . Check 'Em Out' (2002) The Orchid Cancer Appeal [video VHS].

Kraemer S (2000) The fragile male. *BMJ.* **321**: 1609–1612.

LM Research (2005) *Anatomy of a Big Night Out.* London: Portman Group.

Lader D and Meltzer H (2001) *Smoking Related Behaviour and Attitudes, 2000.* London: Office for National Statistics.

Lloyd T and Forrest S (2001) *Boys' and Young Men's Health: literature and practice review. An interim report.* London: HDA.

Lloyd T (1998) *Men's Health: a public health review.* London: Royal College of Nursing.

Lloyd T (2002) *Boys' and Young Men's Health: what works.* London: HDA.

Marwick C (1999) Survey says patients expect little help on sex. *J Am Med Assoc.* **281**: 2173–2174.

McCreary DR and Sadava SW (2001) Gender differences in relationships among perceived attractiveness, life satisfaction, and health in adults as a function of body mass index and perceived weight. *Psychology of Men and Masculinity.* **2**: 108–116.

McCreary DR and Sasse DK (2002) Gender differences in high school students' dieting behavior and their correlates. *International Journal of Men's Health.* **1**: 195–213.

Meyer-Weitz A, Reddy P, Van Den Borne HW, Kok G and Pieterson J (2003) Determinants of multi-partner behaviour of male patients with sexually transmitted infections. *International Journal of Men's Health.* **2**: 149–162.

Men's Health Forum (MHF) (2004) *Getting it Sorted: a policy programme for men's health.* London: MHF.

Men's Health Forum (MHF) (2006) *Mind Your Head: men, boys and mental wellbeing.* National Men's Health Week 2006 Policy Report. London: MHF.

Naidoo J and Wills J (2000) *Health Promotion: foundations for practice.* 2nd ed. London: Baillière Tindall.

National Audit Office (2001) *Tackling Obesity in England.* London: The Stationery Office.

National Lottery Act 1998. London: HMSO.

Newman S (1997) Masculinities, men's bodies and nursing. In: Lawler J (ed.) *The Body in Nursing.* Melbourne: Churchill Livingstone.

O'Brien RK, Hunt K and Hart G (2005) 'It's caveman stuff, but that is to a certain extent how guys still operate': men's accounts of masculinity and help seeking. *Soc Sci Med.* **61**: 503–16.

Office for National Statistics (2006) http://www.statistics.gov.uk/cci/nugget. asp?id=313) [Accessed 29/1/07].

Office for National Statistics (2001) *Psychiatric Morbidity among Adults 2000.* London: ONS.

Pearson S (2003) Promoting sexual health services to young men: findings from focus group discussions. *J Fam Plan Reprod Health Care.* **29**: 194–198.

Pollard J (2007) Working with men via the internet. In: White AK and Pettifer M (eds) *Hazardous Waist: tackling male weight problems.* Oxford: Radcliffe.

Pringle A and Sayers P (2004) It's a goal! Basing a community psychiatric nursing service in a local football stadium. *J R Soc Health.* **124**: 234–238.

Prochaska JO and Velicer WF (1997) The transtheoretical model of health behavior change. *Am J Health Promot.* **12**: 38–48.

Richardson CA and Rabiee F (2001) A question of access: an exploration of the factors that influence the health of young males aged 15 to 19 living in Corby and their use of health care services. *Health Educ J.* **60**: 3–16.

Roe S (2005) *Home Office Statistical Bulletin – Drug Misuse Declared: Findings from the 2004/05 British Crime Survey, England and Wales.* London: Home Office.

Robertson S (2003) Men managing health. *Men's Health J.* **2**: 111–113.

Royal College of Physicians (2004) *Storing Up Problems: the medical case for a slimmer nation*. London: Royal College of Physicians.

Royster M, Richmond A, Eng E and Margolis L (2006) Hey brother, how's your health? A focus group analysis of the health and health-related concerns of African American men in a Southern City in the United States. *Men and Masculinities*. **8**: 389–390.

Saltonstall R (1993) Healthy bodies, social bodies: men's and women's concepts and practices of health in everyday life. *Soc Sci Med*. **36**: 7–14.

Social Exclusion Unit (2003) *Mental Health and Social Exclusion – consultation document, May 2003*. London: SEU.

Spurlock M (2004) *Super Size Me* (DVD). Tartan Video.

Teenage Pregnancy Unit (1999) *Teenage Pregnancy*. London: Social Exclusion Unit.

Teenage Pregnancy Unit (2000) *Guidance for Developing Contraception and Sexual Health Advice Services to Reach Boys and Young Men*. London: DoH.

Teenage Pregnancy Unit (2007) *Teenage Conception Statistics for England 1998–2005*. http://www.everychildmatters.gov.uk/_files/9E0C1F27DA3ED03D6D2E145891 A9A9BD.doc [Accessed 20/4/07].

Tones K and Green J (2004) *Health Promotion: planning and strategies*. London: Sage Publications.

Tones K, Tilford S and Robinson Y (1994) *Health Education – Effectiveness and Efficiency*. 2nd ed. London: Chapman and Hall.

Tudiver F and Talbot Y (1999) Why men don't seek help? Family physicians' perspectives on health-seeking behaviour in men. *J Fam Pract*. **43**: 475–480.

UK Collaborative Group for HIV and STI Surveillance (2004) *Focus on Prevention: HIV and other Sexually Transmitted Infections in the United Kingdom in 2003*. London: HPA.

Verrinder A and Denner BJ (2000) The success of men's health nights and health sessions. *Aust J Rural Health*. **8**: 81–86.

Visser R de and Smith JA (2006) Mister in-between: a case study of masculine identity and health-related behaviour. *J Health Psychol*. **11**: 685–695.

Vonnegut K (1991) *Slaughterhouse 5*. London: Vintage.

Walker BM and Kushner S (1997) *Boys: understanding boys' sexual health education and its implications for attitude change*. Norwich: Centre for Applied Research in Education.

White AK (2001) *Report on the Scoping Study on Men's Health*. London: DoH.

White AK (2006a) Men and mental wellbeing: encouraging gender sensitivity. Personal perspective. *Mental Health Review*. **11**(4): 3–6.

White AK (2006b) Men's health in the 21st Century. *International Journal of Men's Health*. **5**: 1–17.

White AK and Banks I (2004) Help seeking in men and the problems of late diagnosis. In: Kirby RS, Carson CC, Kirby MG and Farah RN (eds) *Men's Health*. 2nd ed. London: Martin Dunitz.

White A and Cash K (2003) *The State of Men's Health Across 17 European Countries*. Brussels: European Men's Health Forum.

White AK and Cash K (2004) The state of men's health in Western Europe. *Journal of Men's Health and Gender*. **1**: 60–66.

White AK and Cash K (2005) *Report on the First Phase of the Study on Men's Usage of the Bradford Health of Men Services.* Leeds: Leeds Metropolitan University.

White AK and Holmes M (2006) Patterns of mortality across 44 countries among men and women aged 15–44. *Journal of Men's Health and Gender.* 3(2): 139–151.

White AK and Pettifer M (2007) *Hazardous Waist: tackling male weight problems.* Oxford: Radcliffe.

Wilkinson R and Marmot M (2003) *Social Determinants of Health: the solid facts.* 2nd ed. Copenhagen: WHO.

Wizemann TM and Pardue ML (2001) *Exploring the Biological Contributions to Human Health: does sex matter?* Washington, DC: Institute of Medicine.

World Health Organization (1986) *Ottawa Charter for Health Promotion, 1986.* Geneva: WHO.

Index